Saliva and Oral Health

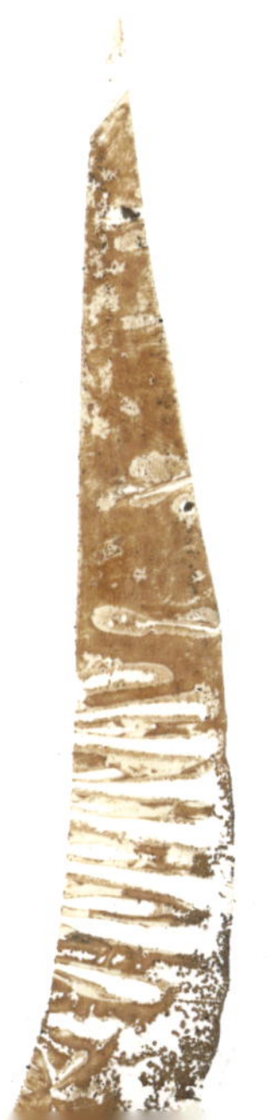

Saliva and Oral Health

SECOND EDITION

Edited by

W. M. Edgar,* DDSc, PhD, BDS, BSc, FDSRCS(Eng)
D. M. O'Mullane,** PhD(NUI), BDS, FDSRCS(Ed), FFDRCSI

**Professsor of Dental Science, School of Dentistry, The University of Liverpool, Liverpool, UK*
***Professor of Preventive and Paediatric Dentistry and Director of Oral Health Services Research Centre, University Dental School and Hospital, Cork, Ireland*

Published by the British Dental Association
64 Wimpole Street, London W1M 8AL

First edition 1990
Second edition 1996
Reprinted 1999

ISBN 0 904588 47 5

Printed and bound in Great Britain by
Thanet Press Limited, Margate

Preface

Since the publication of the first edition of *Saliva and Dental Health* in 1990, knowledge of the secretion, composition and functions of saliva, and especially of its clinical importance in dental and oral health, has expanded dramatically. Of practical importance is the increasing realisation of the impact on the one hand of salivary hypofunction, with the consequent loss of the protective and other functions of saliva, and on the other hand, salivary stimulation, with resulting beneficial effects in reducing the potential for tooth demineralisation and (in conjunction with fluoride) remineralisation. The success of the first edition, which ran to almost 10,000 copies world-wide, gave us confidence to embark upon a second edition, which would update and expand much of the material, and whose broader emphasis would be reflected in a change in the title to include oral and not just dental health.

As with the previous book, the readership was intended, in the main, to be the progressive and inquisitive practitioner, looking for ways of broadening the approach to general dental practice. No less important, however, has been the undergraduate and postgraduate student. For both of these groups, we have aimed to provide a more comprehensive and coherent account while maintaining a high degree of clinical relevance. This has necessitated the introduction of new material as well as the condensation of topics which received perhaps undue emphasis previously. In parallel, the visual and graphic impact has been enhanced and given a more consistent format.

The first edition was the result of an edited transcription of a series of panel discussions led by an expert in each topic. This process gave rise to separate chapters which were not therefore attributable to individual authors. A different approach was taken on this occasion, and selected authors were asked to provide a manuscript incorporating a more or less radical revision of the previous chapters. Each chapter is therefore attributed to one or more author and is substantially based on the author's original manuscript. However, to ensure a degree of continuity and comprehensiveness and to avoid excessive overlaps, the authors gathered together for two days to present their papers verbally and to discuss each chapter in turn. This process resulted in considerably less need for original work by the editors, but nonetheless led to a text which represents a consensus of world experts' opinion.

The editors wish to acknowledge again the contribution made to the first edition by those who participated in the discussions. Their work provided the basis for the first edition, and a starting point for the chapters of the second edition. We reprint the list of contributors, several of whom became chapter authors in the new edition.

The editors acknowledge also the sponsorship of the Wm Wrigley Jr Company in arranging the meeting of authors, prior to the meeting of the International Association for Dental Research in Singapore, June 1995, and in supporting publication costs. Thanks are due also to Pauline Tamplin and Sarah Bradford at Bullet Communications for keeping the project on track, and to Colette Spicer of University College Cork who verified the references.

W. M. Edgar and D. M. O'Mullane
February, 1996

Preface to the First Edition

This book arises from a 2-day Consensus Meeting of selected, world renowned experts on saliva and salivation who were gathered together under the auspices of the University of Cork and supported by thc Wm Wrigley Jr Company to discuss the role of saliva in dental health, and practical aspects of salivary stimulation for clinical dentistry, and especially preventive dentistry of the future. The programme was planned by Dr Colin Dawes, who also selected the participants. The meeting was held in a magnificent castle in a beautiful corner of Ireland on the shores of Loch Corib, reputed to be one of the finest fishing lakes in the world. The meeting was chaired by two major figures in dental research, both of them having held the office of President of the International Association for Dental Research. It is particularly fitting that the chairman for the first day was an Irishman. Dr Bill Bowen, formerly at the Royal College of Surgeons of England, London, is now head of the Department of Dental Research, University of Rochester, USA. Dr Bowen recalled the Irish toast — 'The health of the salmon to you: a long life, a full heart and a wet mouth' — and stressed that the purpose of the meeting was to report on how dental practitioners can help their patients by maintaining a wet mouth.

On the other hand, the chairman for the second day of the meeting, referred to the change in perspective of the profession concerning saliva — regarded as a hindrance to restorative techniques until relatively recently. Dr Ernest Newbrun of the University of California, San Francisco, and author of widely-used textbooks on cariology and fluorides, stressed the essential role of saliva in controlling the environment of the teeth, the benefits to be gained by stimulation and the problems experienced by patients with xerostomia.

The papers were presented in an informal manner allowing full and detailed discussion of each point raised, with the chairman taking pains to ensure that practical, clinical aspects were highlighted. The papers and discussion were taped, and the proceedings transcribed before being extensively edited. What remains is presented in this book, with the aim of summarising in a concise and practical way the present knowledge of saliva and its importance for dental health. It is aimed at the general dental practitioner in the interests of his or her continuing training and to promote the preventive aspects of salivary secretion and properties.

The list of contributors and the titles of their papers, together with other invited delegates, is shown on page ix. The papers formed the basis of the relevant chapters of this book, but points made by other contributors during the general discussion periods have been incorporated in the chapters, and the text has been extensively simplified and edited. The views expressed in this book do not, therefore, necessarily correspond with those of the presenters of the papers. Nevertheless, without their contributions, to act as a source and template, the chapters could not have been compiled, and the editors wish to express their gratitude for the generous help they have received from the contributors at all stages in the preparation of the book.

W. M. Edgar and D. M. O'Mullane
May, 1990

Contributors

Dr William H. Bowen, PhD, BDS, Professor and Chair, Department of Dental Research, University of Rochester, School of Medicine and Dentistry, Rochester, New York, USA.

Dr Colin Dawes, PhD, BSc, BDS, Professor of Oral Biology, Department of Oral Biology, University of Manitoba, Winnipeg, Manitoba, Canada.

Professor W. M. Edgar, PhD, BDS, BSc, DDSc, Professor of Dental Science, School of Dentistry, The University of Liverpool, Liverpool, UK.

Dr D. I. Hay, PhD, Head, Department of Biochemistry, Forsyth Dental Center, Boston, Massachusetts, USA.

Dr Susan M. Higham, BSc, PhD, FIBiol, Lecturer in Oral Biology, School of Dentistry, The University of Liverpool, UK.

Professor V. Leontiev, Doctor of Medical Science, Professor of Dentistry, Professor of Biochemistry General Director, Joint-Stock Company Stomatologia, Moscow, Russia.

Professor D. M. O'Mullane, PhD (NUI), BDS, FDSRCS (Ed), FFDRCSI, Head, Department of Preventive and Paediatric Dentistry, Dental School and Hospital, Cork, Ireland.

Professor J. M. ten Cate, PhD, Professor of Experimental Preventive Dentistry, Department of Cariology and Endodontology, Academic Centre for Dentistry Amsterdam (ACTA), Amsterdam, The Netherlands.

Professor L. M. Sreebny, PhD, DDS, MS, Department of Oral Biology and Pathology, Health Sciences Center, State University of New York at Stony Brook, Stony Brook, New York, USA.

Dr Peter Smith, PhD, BSc, Lecturer in Oral Biology, School of Dentistry, The University of Liverpool, UK.

Dr Helen Whelton, BDS, PhD, NUI, Deputy Director of Oral Health Services Research Centre, University Dental School and Hospital, Cork, Ireland.

Contributors to the First Edition

Dr William H. Bowen, PhD, BDS, Professor and Chair, Department of Dental Research, University of Rochester, School of Medicine and Dentistry, Rochester, New York, USA.

Dr Colin Dawes, PhD, BSc, BDS, Professor of Oral Biology, Department of Oral Biology, University of Manitoba, Winnipeg, Manitoba, Canada. (Physiological factors influencing salivary flow rate and composition.)

Dr G. H. Dibdin, PhD, BSc, MSc, Research Scientist, Medical Research Council Dental Group, Dental School, University of Bristol, Bristol, UK.

Professor W. M. Edgar, DDSc, PhD, BDS, BSc, FDSRCS(Eng), Professor of Dental Science, School of Dentistry, The University of Liverpool, Liverpool, UK.

Dr J. D. B. Featherstone, PhD, MSc, Professor, Department of Restorative Dentistry, University of California at San Francisco, San Francisco, California, USA. (Role of saliva in demineralisation and remineralisation of teeth.)

Dr Norman Fleming, Professor, Department of Oral Biology, University of Manitoba, Winnipeg, Manitoba, Canada. (Secretory mechanisms of salivary glands and their manipulation.)

Professor Dorothy A. M. Geddes, PhD, BDS, FDS, MS, Head, Oral Biology Group, Glasgow Dental School, Glasgow, UK. (Effects of saliva on plaque pH.)

Dr D. I. Hay, PhD, Head, Department of Biochemistry, Forsyth Dental Center, Boston, Massachusetts, USA. (The functions of salivary proteins.)

Dr I. Kleinberg, PhD, DDS, DSc, Professor and Chairman, Department of Oral Biology and Pathology, School of Dental Medicine, State University of New York, Stony Brook, New York, USA.

Dr F. Lagerlöf, PhD, DDS, Odont Dr, Head Clinical Research Centre, School of Dentistry, Karolinska Institutet, Huddinge, Sweden. (Salivary clearance and its effect on oral health.)

Dr M. Joost Larsen, Odont Dr, Associate Professor, Department of Oral Anatomy, Dental Pathology and Operative Dentistry, Royal Dental College, Aarhus, Denmark. (Calculus, caries and salivary saturation with calcium phosphates.)

Dr E. Newbrun, PhD, BDS, MS, DMD, Odont Dr (Hon), Professor of Oral Biology and Periodontology, Division of Oral Biology, Department of Stomatology, Unversity of California, San Francisco, California, USA.

Professor D. M. O'Mullane, PhD (NUI), BDS, FDSRCS (Ed), FFDRCSI, Head, Department of Preventive and Paediatric Dentistry, Dental School and Hospital, Cork, Eire.

Dr J. S. van der Hoeven, PhD, Institute of Preventive and Community Dentistry, University of Nijmegen, Nijmegen, Holland. (Effects of saliva on plaque microbiology.)

Contents

	Preface	v
	Preface to the First Edition	vi
	Contributors	viii
	Contributors to the First Edition	ix
1	Introduction: the anatomy and physiology of the salivary glands *Helen Whelton*	1
2	Mechanisms of secretion by salivary glands *Peter M Smith*	9
3	Factors influencing salivary flow rate and composition *Colin Dawes*	27
4	Xerostomia: diagnosis, management and clinical complications *Leo M Sreebny*	43
5	Clearance of substances from the oral cavity — implications for oral health *Colin Dawes*	67
6	Saliva and the control of plaque pH *Michael Edgar and Susan M Higham*	81
7	Salivary influences on the oral microflora *William H Bowen*	95
8	The functions of salivary proteins *Donald I Hay and William H Bowen*	105
9	The role of saliva in mineral equilibrium — caries and calculus formation *Bob ten Cate*	123
	Index	137

1

Introduction: The Anatomy and Physiology of Salivary Glands

Helen Whelton

Saliva is the glandular secretion which constantly bathes the teeth and the oral mucosa. It is constituted by the secretions of the three paired major salivary glands, the parotid, submandibular and sublingual, the minor salivary glands and the gingival fluid.

The presence of saliva is vital to the maintenance of healthy oral tissues. Severe reduction of salivary output not only results in a rapid deterioration in oral health but also has a detrimental impact on quality of life for the sufferer. Patients suffering from dry mouth experience difficulty with eating, swallowing, speech, retention of dentures, taste alteration, oral hygiene, trauma and ulceration of the oral mucosa, a burning sensation of the mucosa, oral infections including Candida and rapidly progressive dental caries. Dry mouth or xerostomia is becoming increasingly common in developed countries where adults are living longer. Polypharmacy is very common amongst the older adult population and many of the commonly prescribed drugs cause a reduction in salivary flow. Xerostomia also occurs in Sjögren's syndrome which is not an uncommon condition. In addition to specific diseases of the salivary glands salivary flow is usually reversibly or irreversibly, severely impaired following radiotherapy in the head and neck area for cancer treatment in both children and adults of all ages. Clearly, xerostomia is a problem which faces an increasingly large proportion of the population. An understanding of saliva and its role in oral health will help to promote an awareness amongst health care workers of the problem, its prevention and treatment.

Functions of saliva

The complexity of this oral fluid is perhaps best appreciated by the consideration of its many and varied functions.The functions of saliva are largely protective; however it also has other functions. Table 1.1

provides an overview of many of these functions. More detail is provided in subsequent chapters as indicated.

Table 1.1 Functions of saliva

Fluid/Lubricant	Coats mucosa and helps to protect against mechanical, thermal and chemical irritation. Assists smooth air flow, speech and swallowing (Ch. 8)
Ion reservoir	Solution supersaturated with ions facilitates remineralisation of the teeth (Ch. 9)
Buffer	Helps to neutralise plaque pH after eating, thus reducing time for demineralisation (Ch. 6)
Cleansing	Clears food and aids swallowing (Ch. 3 & 5)
Antimicrobial actions	Specific (eg sIgA) and non specific (eg Lysozyme, Lactoferrin and Sialoperoxidase) anti-microbial mechanisms help control the oral microflora (Ch. 7 & 8)
Agglutination	Aggregation and accelerated clearance of bacterial cells (Ch. 7)
Pellicle formation	Protective diffusion barrier formed on enamel from salivary proteins
Digestion	Due to the presence of the enzyme amylase, starchy food debris on the teeth is broken down (Ch. 8)
Taste	Saliva acts as a solvent thus allowing interaction of foodstuff with taste buds to facilitate taste (Ch 8)
Excretion	As the oral cavity is technically outside the body, substances which are secreted in saliva are excreted. This is a very inefficient excretory pathway as reabsorption may occur further down the intestinal tract.
Water balance	Under conditions of dehydration, salivary flow is reduced, dryness of the mouth and information from osmoreceptors are translated into decreased urine production and increased drinking (integrated by the hypothalamus, Ch. 3)

The type of secretion varies according to gland. The parotid secretion is serous or watery in consistency, that from the submandibular and sublingual is much more viscous due to its glycoprotein content. The histology of the gland therefore varies according to gland type.

Anatomy and histology

All of the salivary glands develop in a similar way. An ingrowth of epithelium from the stomatodeum extends deeply into the ectomesenchyme and branches profusely to form all the working parts of the gland. The surrounding ectomesenchyme then differentiates to form the connective tissue component of the gland ie the capsule and fibrous septa that divide the gland into lobes. These developments take place between 4 and 12 weeks of embryonic life, the parotids being the first and the sublingual and minor salivary glands being the last to develop. Figure 1.1 shows some of the relations of both the parotid and submandibular glands.

The parotids are the largest salivary glands. They are wedge shaped with the base of the wedge lying superficially covered by skin, superficial fascia and the parotid capsule. They are situated in front of the ear and behind the ramus of the mandible. The apex of the wedge is the deepest part of the gland. The gland is intimately associated with the peripheral branches of the facial nerve (CN VII). This relationship is particularly noticeable when an inferior alveolar nerve block is inadvertently administered too high up in a child. In this situation the anaesthetic is delivered into the parotid gland and the facial nerve is anaesthetised thus resulting in an alarming appearance of a drooping eyelid which is of course temporary.

The parotid duct is thick walled, formed by the union of the ductules which drain the lobules of the glands. It emerges at the anterior border of the gland on the surface of the masseter and hooks medially over its anterior border. It can be felt at this point by moving a finger over the muscle with the jaw clenched. The duct opens into the oral cavity in a papilla opposite the second upper molar tooth.

The submandibular gland is variable in size but about half the size of the parotid. Its superficial part is wedged between the body of the mandible and the mylohyoid muscle (which forms the floor of the mouth). The gland hooks around the sharply defined posterior border of the mylohyoid muscle and its smaller deep part lies above mylohyoid in the floor of the mouth. The thin walled duct runs forward in the angle between the side of the tongue and mylohyoid. It opens into the floor of the mouth underneath the anterior part of the tongue, on the summit

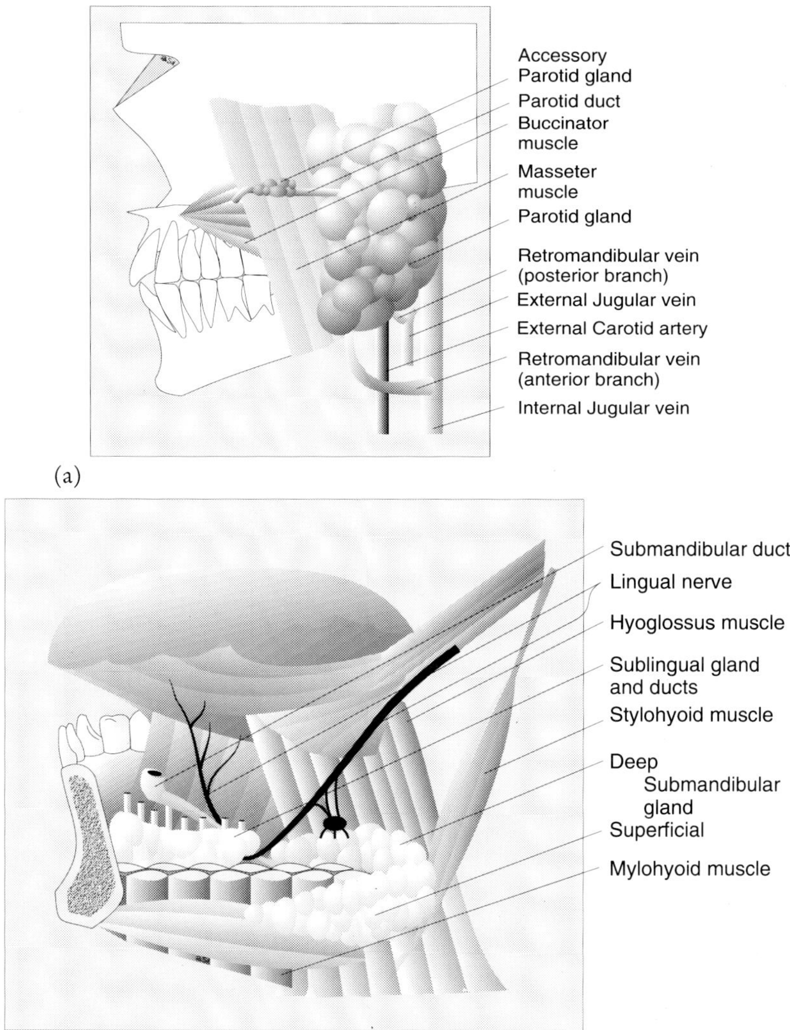

Fig. 1.1 Some relations of (a) the parotid and (b) the submandibular glands

of the sublingual papilla lateral to the lingual fraenum. The secretions are a mixture of mucous and serous fluids.

The sublingual is the smallest of the paired major salivary glands being about one fifth the size of the submandibular. It is situated in the floor of the mouth beneath the sublingual folds of mucous membrane. Numerous small ducts (8–20) open into the mouth on the summit of the sublingual fold. It is predominantly a mucous gland.

Minor salivary glands are situated on the tongue, palate and buccal and labial mucosa. They are small mucosal glands with primarily a mucous secretion.

Structure of salivary glands

The working parts of the salivary glandular tissue (fig. 1.2) consist of the secretory end pieces (acini) and the branched ductal system. In serous glands (eg the parotids) the cells in the end piece are arranged in a roughly spherical form. In mucous glands they tend to be arranged in a tubular configuration with a larger central lumen. In both types of gland the intercellular spaces between the cells in the end piece open into the lumen and this is the start of the ductal system. There are three types of duct present in all salivary glands. The fluid first passes through the intercalated ducts which have low cuboidal epithelium and a narrow lumen. From there the secretions enter the striated ducts which are lined by more columnar cells with many mitochondria. Finally, the saliva passes through the excretory ducts where the cell type is cuboidal until the terminal part which is lined with stratified squamous epithelium.

End pieces may contain mucous cells, serous cells or a mixture of both. A salivary gland can consist of a varied mixture of these types of

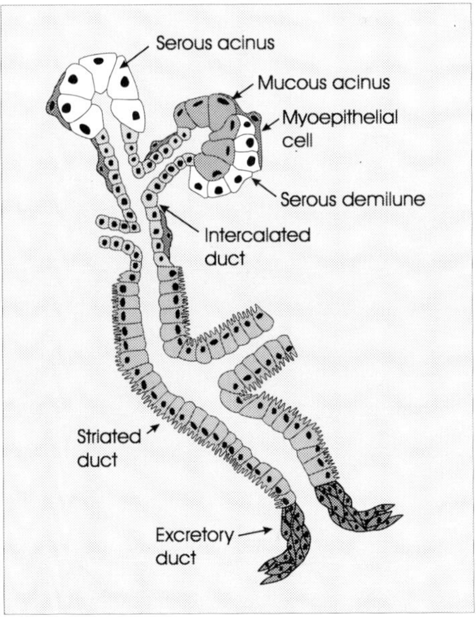

Fig. 1.2 Structure of salivary gland.

end pieces. In mixed glands, the mucous acini are capped by a serous demilune. In addition, myoepithelial cells surround the end piece, their function being to assist in propelling the secretion into the ductal system. The gland and its specialised nerve and blood supply are supported by a connective tissue stroma.

Formation of saliva

The fluid formation in salivary glands occurs in the end pieces (acini) where serous cells produce a watery seromucous secretion and mucous cells produce a viscous mucin rich secretion. These secretions arise by the formation from blood in capillaries of interstitial fluid which is then modified by the end piece cells to produce the fluid which is secreted into the lumen. From the lumen it passes through the ductal system where it is further modified. Most of the modification occurs in the striated ducts where ion exchange takes place and the secretion is changed from an isotonic solution to a hypotonic one. The composition of saliva is further modified in the excretory ducts before it is finally secreted into the mouth (see Chapter 2 for a detailed account of saliva secretory mechanisms).

Nerve supply

The glands receive both parasympathetic and sympathetic nerve supplies. Secretion is controlled mainly by parasympathetic impulses from the salivary nuclei which are located approximately at the juncture of the pons and the medulla and are excited by both taste and mechanical stimuli from the tongue and other areas of the mouth via afferent sensory fibres. Salivation can also be stimulated or inhibited by impulses arriving in the salivary nuclei from higher centres of the central nervous system. For example, in stressful situations dry mouth sometimes occurs not as a result of any direct sympathetic inhibition as was previously thought, but rather as a result of the inhibitory effect of higher centres on salivary nuclei.

Reflexes originating in the stomach and upper intestines also stimulate salivation. For example, when very irritating foods are swallowed or when a person is nauseated the saliva serves to dilute or neutralise the irritating substances.

Sympathetic stimulation can also increase salivary flow to a moderate extent but much less so than parasympathetic stimulation. Sympathetic impulses are more likely to influence salivary composition by increasing exocytosis from certain cells. The sympathetic nerves originate from the superior cervical ganglia and then travel along the blood vessels to the salivary glands. Salivary composition may also be influenced by hormones such as androgens, oestrogens, glucocorticoids and peptide hormones.

Blood supply

The blood supply to the glands also influences secretion. An extensive blood supply is required for the rapid secretion of saliva. There is a concentration of capillaries around the striated ducts where ionic exchange takes place whilst a lesser density supplies the terminal secretory systems. The process of salivation indirectly dilates the blood vessels thus providing increased nutrition as needed. Salivary secretion is usually accompanied by a large increase in blood flow.

Physiology

Composition

The composition of saliva varies according to many factors including the gland type from which it is secreted. The composition of whole saliva is of interest as this is the fluid which constantly bathes the teeth. The average composition of a sample of mixed saliva is shown in Table 1.2.

Flow rate

Salivary flow rates exhibit both diurnal and seasonal variation with peaks in mid afternoon and higher flow rates in the Spring than in the Autumn. Normal salivary flow rates are in the region of 0.3 ml/min when unstimulated and 1.5–2.0 ml/min when stimulated, although both rates have wide normal ranges (see Chapter 3). Approximately 0.5 litres of saliva is secreted per day, of which 25% comes from the submandibular salivary glands and 66% from the parotids. During sleep, flow rate is negligible.

Many drugs used frequently for the treatment of common conditions such as for example, hypertension, depression and allergies (to mention but a few) also influence salivary flow rate and composition. Factors influencing salivary composition are considered in more detail in Chapter 3.

The determination of a patients salivary flow rate is a simple procedure. Both resting and stimulated flow rates can be measured and changes in flow can be monitored over time. Salivary flow and measurement is considered further in Chapter 3. Other clinical investigations of salivary function such as sialography and scintiscanning require referral for specialist evaluation.

Table 1.2 The average composition of mixed human saliva and normal values for plasma

		Unstimulated (%)	Stimulated (%)
Water		99.4	99.5
Solids		0.6	0.5
Specific gravity	1.002–1.008		
Average pH	6.7		
pH range	6.2–7.6		
		Saliva (mM)	**Plasma (mM)**
Inorganic			
	Ca^{2+}	1–2	2.5
	Mg^{2+}	0.2–0.5	1.0
	Na^+	6–26	140
	K^+	14–32	4
	NH_4^+	1–7	0.03
	$H_2PO_4^-$ & HPO_4^{2-}	2–23	2
	Cl^-	17–29	103
	HCO_3^-	2–30	27
	F^-	0.0005–0.005	0.001
	SN^-	0.1–2.0	—
Organic			
	Urea (adults)	2–6	5
	Urea (children)	1–2	—
	Uric acid	0.2	3
	Amino acids (free)	1–2	2
	Glucose (free)	0.05	5
	Lactate	0.1	1
	Fatty acids (mg/l)	10	3000
Macromolecules (mg/l)			
	Proteins	1400–2000	70 000
	Glycoprotein sugars	110–300	1400
	Amylase	380	—
	Lysozyme	109	—
	Peroxidase	3	—
	IgA	194	1300
	IgG	14	13 000
	IgM	2	1000
	Lipid	20–30	5500

Further reading

Bradley R M. Salivary secretion. In *Essentials of oral physiology*, 2nd ed. pp 161–186. St Louis: Mosby, 1995.

Cole A S, Eastoe J E. The oral environment. In *Biochemistry and oral biology*, 2nd ed. pp 475–489. Bristol: Wright, 1988.

Ten Cate A R. Salivary glands. In *Oral histology development, structure and function*, 3rd ed. pp 312–340. St Louis: Mosby, 1989.

2

Mechanisms of Secretion by Salivary Glands

Peter M Smith

In recent years, understanding of stimulus-secretion coupling and secretory mechanisms has developed far from the black box concept as the tools to open the box and look inside have become available. The application of three new technologies in particular to salivary gland research has provided much of the information currently enjoyed and promises to provide more in the future.

1 Molecular biology techniques have been employed to detail the mechanisms of protein synthesis, segregation and storage.

2 Various manifestations of the patch-clamp technique have allowed direct identification of the ion channels responsible for electrolyte and ultimately fluid secretion. The patch-clamp technique has also been used to measure the tiny changes in plasma membrane capacitance associated with fusion of secretory vesicles and exocytosis.

3 Microfluorimetric measurement of intracellular Ca^{2+} concentration in single cells, and in particular imaging of such data, have revealed spatial and temporal aspects of Ca^{2+} mobilisation which may have a critical bearing on the mechanisms of electrolyte and fluid secretion.

The detailed information provided by these powerful techniques may lead beyond an appreciation of how salivary glands function under normal conditions towards understanding salivary gland dysfunction associated with disease. Patch-clamp and molecular biology techniques in combination have already successfully identified the defect in Cl^- transport which causes cystic fibrosis. Similar research in progress at present could help to elucidate the cellular and molecular basis of xerostomia and Sjögren's syndrome in particular.

Saliva is a complex fluid with unique lubricant, antibacterial and digestive properties. In addition, stimulated saliva is a powerful buffer which plays a crucial role in limiting the pH change following acid production by plaque bacteria. Salivary acinar cells produce the macromolecules which give saliva its unique properties and the acinar and duct cells combine to produce a hypotonic fluid vehicle to carry the salivary macromolecules into the mouth. Fluid secretion and macromolecule secretion occur by separate processes. Both are under the control of the autonomic nervous system, both are stimulated by the presence of food in the mouth. Parasympathetic nerves release acetylcholine (ACh) and stimulate fluid secretion, sympathetic nerves release noradrenaline (NA) and stimulate protein secretion (fig. 2.1).

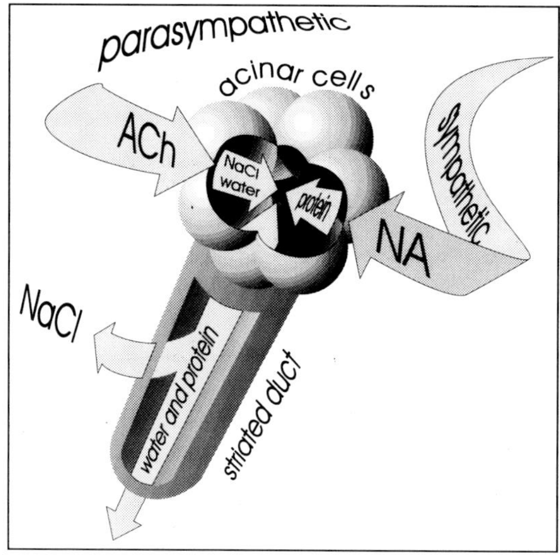

Fig. 2.1 Salivary secretion.

The neural control of salivation is outlined in figure 2.2. The afferent pathways for taste are via the facial and glossopharyngeal nerves to a solitary nucleus in the medulla. There is also an input from higher centres in response to smell, sight etc. The parasympathetic efferent pathways for the sublingual and submandibular glands are from the facial nerve via the submandibular ganglion; for the parotid gland they are from the glossopharyungeal nerve via the otic ganglion. The sympathetic post ganglionic pathways are from the cervical ganglion of

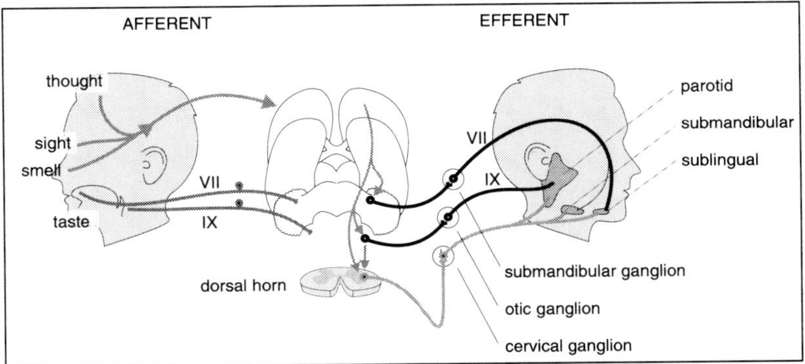

Fig. 2.2 Neural control of salivation

the sympathetic chain. The neurotransmitter is the first messenger in the communication pathway between nerves and secretion. Neurotransmitters exert their activity at the cell membrane; they cannot reach inside the cell to activate intracellular processes but rather they communicate with intracellular second messengers which have direct control of the cellular machinery responsible for secretion. In order to understand how secretion occurs and how the secretory process is controlled, we must identify key secretory events, determine which second messengers control these events and link second messenger production back to receptor activation by neurotransmitter.

Fluid and electrolyte secretion

Salivary gland cellular anatomy and transport mechanisms

Salivary glands are largely composed of epithelial cells. Epithelial cells are both structurally and functionally polarised; that is to say that the appearance and behaviour of one end of the cell is very different from that of the other. The ability of the salivary glands to produce a protein rich hypotonic saliva is a direct consequence of epithelial cell polarisation.

One important determinant of epithelial cell polarisation is the plasma membrane, which is divided into two parts (fig. 2.3). The apical (top) membrane faces into the lumen and the basolateral (bottom and sides) membrane faces the gap between adjacent cells (lateral intercellular space) and the blood capillaries. The division between apical and basolateral membranes occurs at the tight junctions which connect adjacent cells at the apical border. One of the functions of the tight junctions may be to prevent mixing of apical and basolateral membrane components. However, the primary function of the tight junctions is to

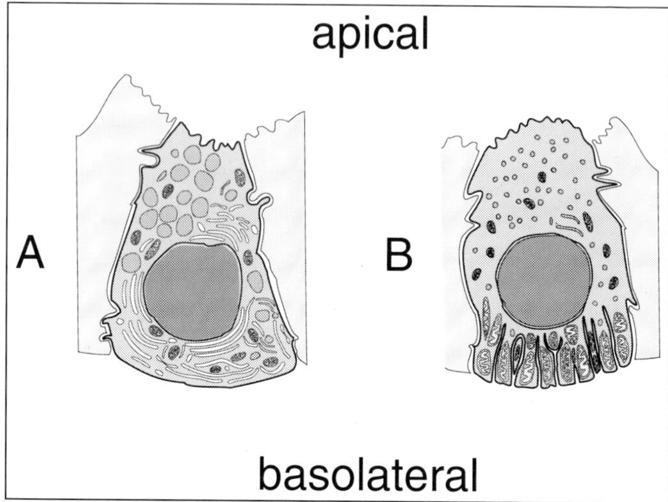

Fig. 2.3 Polarisation in two major epithelial cell types found in salivary glands. (a) Acinar cell showing the presence of secretory vesicles at the apical pole (b) Striated duct cell showing a high density of mitochondria at the basolateral pole

act as a barrier to transepithelial transport. The nature of the barrier presented by the tight junctions depends on the function of the epithelium. In salivary gland striated ducts, the tight junctions restrict the passage of all substances, including water, whereas the acinar cell tight junctions prevent anions moving across the epithelium but allow water and cations, such as Na^+, to pass freely.

Fluid and electrolyte secretion in salivary glands involves transport of salt and water from the blood into the lumen of the salivary gland duct. In order to accomplish this therefore, salt and water must cross the epithelial cell layer (transepithelial transport), either between the cells via the tight junctions (paracellular transport) or across both the basolateral and apical cell membranes (transcellular transport). Paracellular transport is always passive and often down an electrochemical gradient created by the epithelial cells. As plasma membrane lipid is impermeable to any polar molecule, electrolytes require channels or transporters in order to take a transcellular route across the epithelium.

A diagrammatic representation of a gated Na^+ channel is shown in figure 2.4. The channel consists of a hydrophilic central domain which permits the passage of Na^+ when the gate is open surrounded by a hydrophobic domain to allow the channel to sit in the plasma mem-

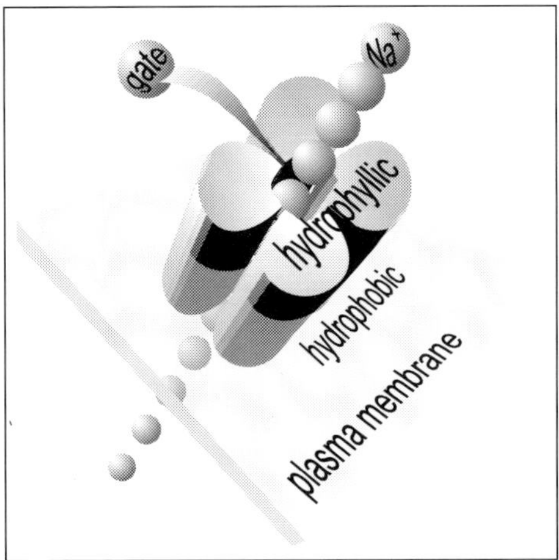

Fig. 2.4 Gated Na^+ channel.

brane. Ion channels can be highly selective (by virtue of their geometry and the presence of fixed surface charges) and also gated. Depending on the type of ion channel, the gate may be opened by for example depolarisation of the membrane potential (voltage operated channels; VOC) or as a direct result of occupancy of a plasma membrane receptor (receptor operated channels; ROC) or following production of some intracellular second messenger (second messenger operated channels; SMOC) The Ca^{2+} activated K^+ and Cl^- channels in salivary acinar cells are examples of second messenger operated channels. Like the tight junctions, movement through channels is always passive, down an electrochemical gradient cells must use active transport mechanisms in order to create electrochemical gradients.

Active transport is accomplished by membrane bound proteins which can utilise metabolic energy, either directly or indirectly to move substrates against their electrochemical gradient. The most widely occurring active transporter is the Na^+/K^+ ATPase (Na^+ pump) which extrudes Na^+ from the cells in exchange for K^+ (fig. 2.5). The Na^+ pump is always found on the basolateral membrane of epithelial cells which explains how part of the functional polarity of epithelial cells is achieved. The Na^+ pump is an example of primary active transport because it uses metabolic energy directly by hydrolysing ATP. One consequence of Na^+ pump activity is that intracellular K^+ is much higher than extracellular K^+, therefore K^+ leaves the cells through K^+ channels and thus creates the membrane potential (which opposes further K^+ efflux). The Na^+ pump also creates an

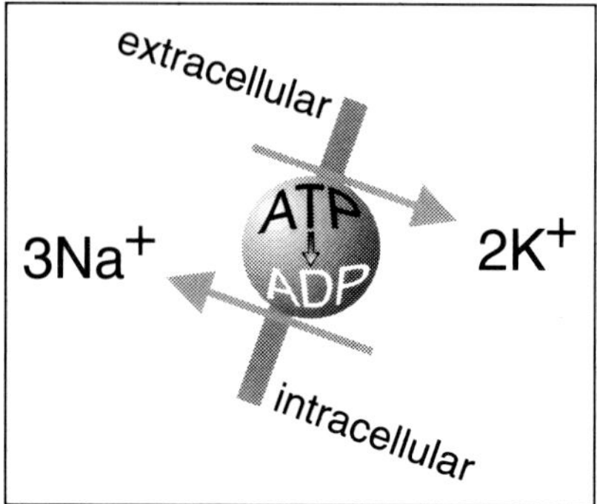

Fig. 2.5 The Na^+ pump hydrolyses ATP in order to extrude Na^+ in exchange for K^+.

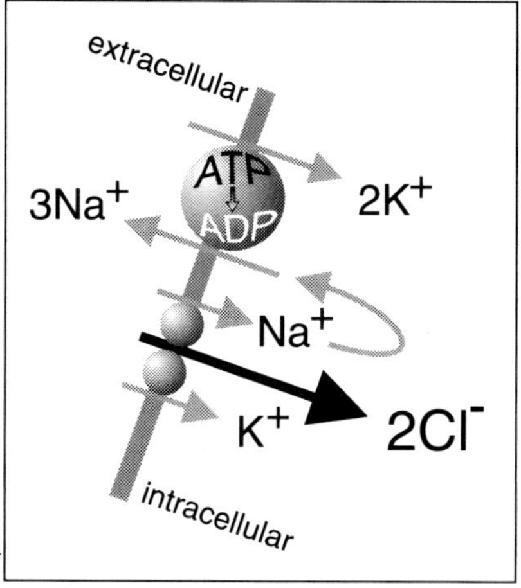

Fig. 2.6 Secondary active Cl^- accumulation driven by the Na^+ gradient.

inwardly directed Na^+ gradient. Both the membrane potential and the Na^+ gradient represent energy sources which can be utilised to drive secondary active transport by cotransport (symport) or countertransport (antiport). A cotransporter will only allow Na^+ to re-enter the cell down its gradient if it brings something (which the cell wants) with it. A countertransporter will only allow Na^+ to re-enter the cell in exchange for something else leaving the cell.

Acinar cells need to increase the intracellular concentration of Cl^- as part of the secretory process, this is achieved by a basolateral $Na^+/K^+/2Cl^-$ cotransporter which uses the energy contained in the Na^+ gradient to concentrate Cl^- within the cell (fig. 2.6).

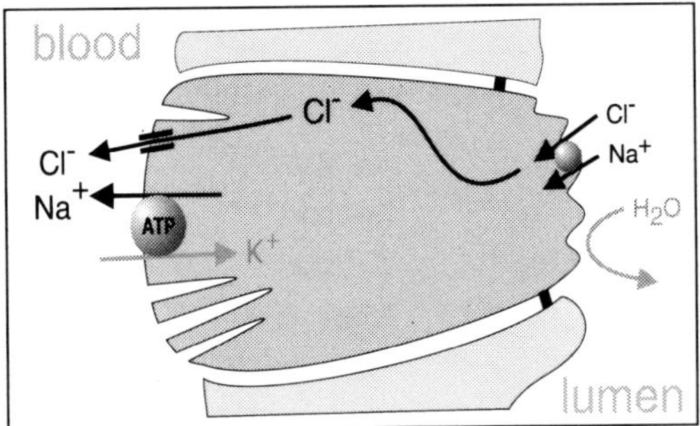

Fig. 2.7 NaCl reabsorbtion by a striated duct cell

The two stage hypothesis

The most straightforward way for the salivary glands to create a hypotonic saliva would be to pump more water than salt from the blood into the salivary ducts. Unfortunately, cells do not have any mechanisms for bulk transport of fluid which do not also involve transport of electrolytes. So the best any cell, including salivary acinar cells, can manage is a secretion isotonic with the blood. A hypotonic saliva *can* be achieved because cells have developed mechanisms for removing ions from the secreted fluid, leaving the water behind. Therefore production of hypotonic saliva is a two stage process. First the acinar cells secrete an isotonic primary saliva and then the striated duct cells actively extract ions to render the saliva progressively more hypotonic as it progresses down the ducts towards the mouth (fig. 2.7).

The infoldings of the basal membrane of the striated duct cells contain many mitochondria which provide ATP to the Na^+ pump which actively extrudes Na^+ back into the blood. Chloride follows passively but water can not because the apical membrane of the striated duct is water impermeable. At low rates of flow, the reabsorptive process can cope with practically all the secreted bicarbonate and most of the secreted NaCl. As flow rates increase, saliva passes through the striated ducts before reabsorption is complete so NaCl and bicarbonate concentrations and the total osmolarity of saliva increase with flow rate (fig. 2.8).

The primary saliva: mechanisms for fluid and electrolyte secretion

Cells cannot produce a hypotonic secretion because fluid transport follows electrolyte transport. Na^+ and Cl^- are transported to the lumen of the acinus; this makes the lumen hypertonic with respect to blood, and water moves by osmosis to redress the balance. If the movement of fluid

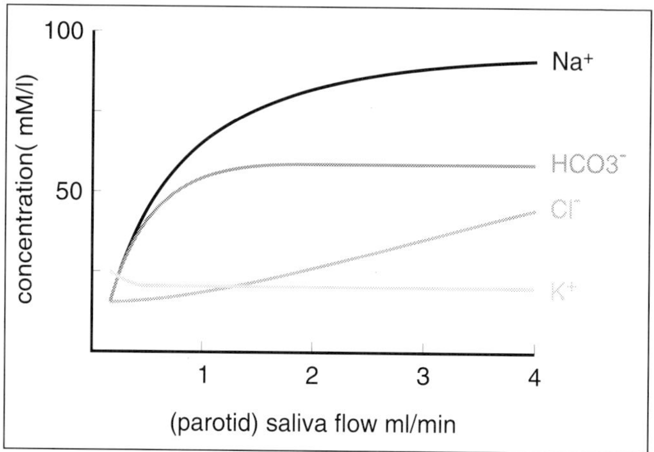

Fig. 2.8 Electrolyte concentration as a function of salivary flow rate. See also Chapter 3

ever caught up with Na^+ and Cl^- transport, there would be no driving force for any further fluid movement. Therefore, the control of primary saliva secretion lies within the mechanisms for Na^+ and Cl^- secretion.

The primary active transport process which underlies practically all bulk solute transport is the ubiquitous Na^+/K^+ ATPase. This creates the Na^+ gradient which energises Cl^- accumulation within the cells by secondary active transport. Under resting conditions Cl^- can not get out of the cell, but when stimulated to secrete, Cl^- channels in the luminal membrane of the acinar cells open to provide an exit for Cl^- which now has a clear pathway across the cell from blood to lumen. Sodium follows Cl^- to preserve electroneutrality and now there is luminal hypertonicity to drive water transport. Thus, Cl^- transport is the key to fluid secretion, the basolateral cotransporter creates the driving force for Cl^- efflux and Cl^- channels act as an on/off switch for secretion. The Cl^- channels themselves are opened by an agonist-evoked increase in $[Ca^{2+}]_i$. The mechanism of fluid secretion in acinar cells is illustrated in figure 2.9. Increased $[Ca^{2+}]_i$ also activates a K^+ channel. This serves to maintain the membrane potential which provides an important part of the driving force for Cl^- efflux.

Bicarbonate secretion

Bicarbonate is reabsorbed along with Na^+ and Cl^- by the salivary gland duct cells and, in resting saliva, HCO_3^- concentration is low; about 1–2mM. Like NaCl concentration, HCO_3^- concentration increases with

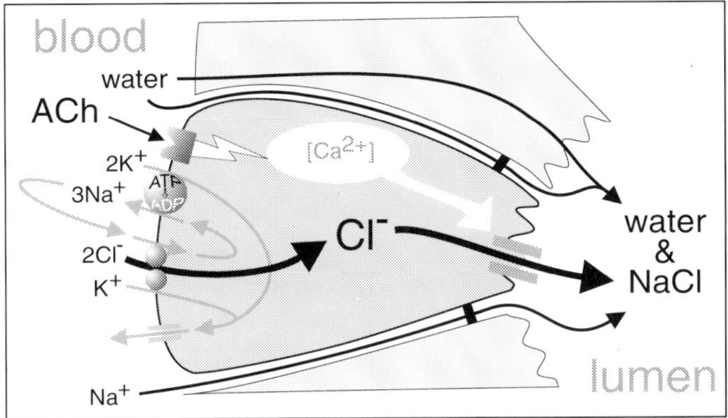

Fig. 2.9 Mechanism of fluid secretion in acinar cells

flow rate, up to 60mM in stimulated saliva. As this maximal salivary HCO_3^- concentration exceeds the plasma HCO_3^- concentration of 24mM, HCO_3^- must be actively secreted by the salivary glands, probably by the acinar cells. The mechanisms by which HCO_3^- is secreted have been less closely studied than those for fluid and electrolytes, but it is thought that the secretory process is similar to that for Cl^- inasmuch as the exit for HCO_3^- from the cells is also driven by membrane potential and is activated by cholinergic agonists. One possibility is that HCO_3^- and Cl^- compete for the same channel (ie the Cl^- channel is also HCO_3^- permeable). Alternatively HCO_3^- might have its own efflux pathway and simply compete with Cl^- for a common driving force.

The concentrating uptake step for HCO_3^- is quite different to that for Cl^-. Intracellular HCO_3^- is derived from the carbonic anhydrase-catalysed hydrolysis of carbon dioxide which diffuses into the cells across the basolateral membrane. Protons are also produced by this reaction, they are extruded from the cell across the basolateral membrane by Na^+/H^+ exchange (countertransport) so that intracellular pH is maintained (fig. 2.10).

Control of fluid secretion: IP_3 and Ca^{2+} as second messengers[1,2]

Cl^- channel activity is regulated by intracellular Ca^{2+} concentration. Cytosolic Ca^{2+} is maintained at very low concentrations (< 100 nM) so that a small increase in concentration can act as an intracellular signal. In response to stimulation, acinar cells mobilise Ca^{2+} from stores held within the cell, supplemented by influx of extracellular Ca^{2+}. The steps between acetylcholine release from nerve terminals and increased intracellular Ca^{2+} have been the focus of much research over the last decade and, as the

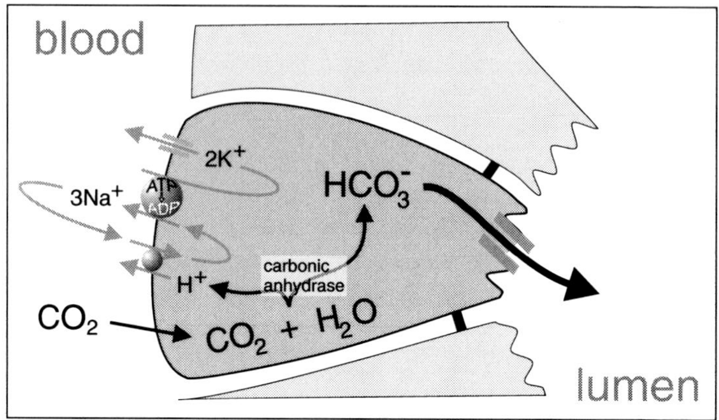

Fig. 2.10 Mechanism of bicarbonate secretion

processes involved have been elucidated, stimulus-secretion coupling has been revealed as a complex and subtle process.

The five basic steps in stimulus-fluid secretion are outlined in figure 2.11. The muscarinic receptors on acinar cells which bind ACh(1) belong to the superfamily of GTPdependent protein (G-protein) coupled receptors having seven membrane-spanning domains. These receptors do not themselves regulate enzyme activity; instead they activate a G-protein so that it may now bind GTP and be converted to an active state(2). The GTP-bound G-protein activates the target enzymes. This G-protein binding step may represent an amplification mechanism because one receptor can activate multiple G-proteins. The G-protein coupled to muscarinic ACh receptors in acinar cells stimulates the enzyme phospholipase-C to cleave phosphoinositol-bis-phosphate (PIP_2) into inositol (1,4,5) trisphosphate (IP_3) and diacylglycerol (DAG)(3). DAG functions as a plasma membrane-bound second messenger but its importance is secondary to that of IP_3 so far as Ca^{2+} mobilisation is concerned. IP_3 is a cytoplasmic second messenger which binds to and activates a Ca^{2+} channel on intracellular Ca^{2+} stores, causing them to release Ca^{2+}(4). As the Ca^{2+} stores empty, Ca^{2+} influx is initiated. The resultant increase in cytosolic Ca^{2+} concentration(5) activates Cl^- channels and give rise to fluid secretion (fig. 2.12).

Pharmacological control of fluid and electrolyte secretion

Fluid and electrolyte secretion may be stimulated by any muscarinic cholinergic agonist. Salivary gland hyposecretion associated with

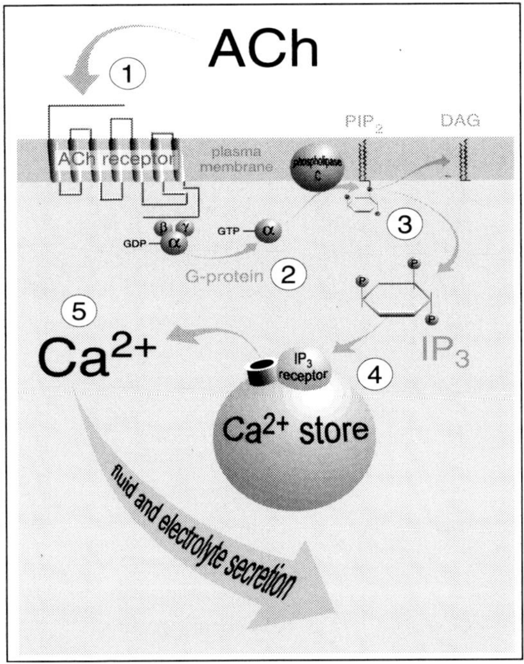

Fig. 2.11 Stimulus-fluid secretion coupling by IP_3 and Ca^{2+} in salivary acinar cells.

Sjogrens syndrome may be treated with topical application of a low dose of pilocarpine. Pilocarpine is a naturally occurring alkaloid (from the leaflets of South American shrubs of the genus Pilocarpus) which has its major action at muscarinic receptors; unlike ACh, pilocarpine is not rapidly metabolised. Therapeutic application of muscarinic agonists is not without side effects (sweating etc.) but these are usually tolerated in preference to dry mouth (see Chapter 4). Saliva production may be blocked by cholinergic receptor antagonists, such as atropine, which compete with ACh for muscarinic receptors and prevent the effects of parasympathetic stimulation on fluid and electrolyte secretion. Other drugs, such as the antipsychotic chlorpromazine, also have anticholinergic actions and can cause hyposecretion.

The increase in cytosolic Ca^{2+} in response to submaximal ACh stimulation is not static but occurs as a series of large, transient increases[4] at a frequency of about once every 5 seconds (fig. 2.13). These transients may be restricted to the luminal pole, which is all that would be required to activate the luminal Cl^- channels.[4] This mechanism is energy efficient

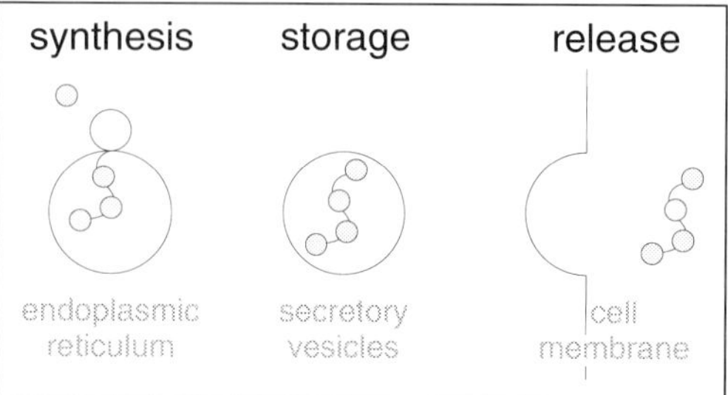

Fig. 2.12 Protein synthesis and release. Proteins are synthesised within membrane-bound structures so that these may fuse with the cell membrane and release their contents

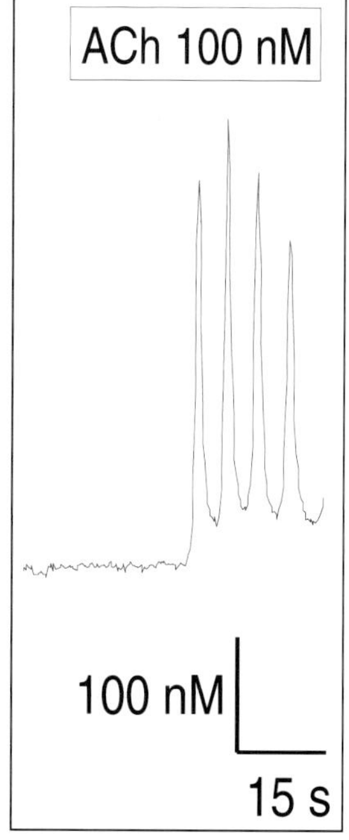

Fig. 2.13 Intracellular [Ca^{2+}] measured in a mouse submandibular cell showing rapid transient increases in response to a low concentration of ACh.

and avoids the toxic effects of cytosolic Ca^{2+} while allowing free control over Cl^- channel activity and hence fluid secretion.

Not all aspects of the Ca^{2+} signalling mechanism have been elucidated. For example, how does the depletion of Ca^{2+} stores stimulate Ca^{2+} influx? Are the Ca^{2+} stores solely within the endoplasmic reticulum or can Ca^{2+} also be released from secretion granules (conveniently situated at the luminal pole)? Finally, other ways of mobilising Ca^{2+} in addition to IP_3 may exist. These questions are the subject of much current research.

Macromolecule secretion

The polypeptides and proteins are synthesised and released by the salivary acinar cells. One of the differences among the major salivary glands is the nature of their protein secretion. Sublingual saliva, produced by mucous acinar cells, is rich in glycoproteins and is, as a consequence, very thick and viscous. The serous acinar cells of the parotid produce mainly salivary amylase and proline rich polypeptides and parotid saliva is thin and watery. The submandibular glands contain a mix of mucous and serous acini which generate an intermediate saliva. Whatever the protein, when it is fully synthesised, it will be much too large to cross the cell membrane. Therefore it must be synthesised and stored within a membrane-bound structure so that it may be released from the cell by exocytosis.

Secretory mechanisms

Synthesis of secretory proteins begins with gene transcription and manufacture of messenger RNA to carry the sequence information from the nucleus to ribosomes in the cytoplasm. Secretory proteins start with a signal sequence which targets the developing polypeptide to the endoplasmic reticulum (ER) where it is N-glycosylated and folded into the correct three-dimensional structure. Small membrane vesicles carry proteins from the ER through several layers of the golgi apparatus for additional processing and packaging for export. Proteins move by default onwards from the ER; those destined to remain in the cell contain specific retention sequences to segregate them from secretory proteins. Secretory proteins are concentrated within golgi condensing-vacuoles and stored in secretory vesicles. As these mature they are transported close to the apical membrane. In response to a secretory stimulus, secretory vesicles fuse with the plasma membrane and discharge their contents outside the cell.

Control of protein secretion: cAMP as a second messenger

The secretory process may be divided into three stages (see fig. 2.12). Synthesis, packaging, and storage and release. Each of these stages is regulated by phosphorylation of target proteins which is brought about by a protein kinase such as cyclic adenosine monophosphate

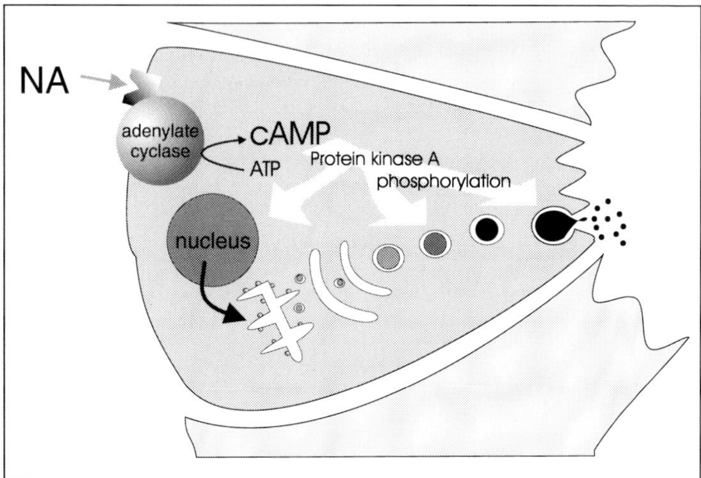

Fig. 2.14 Protein synthesis and release in acinar cells

(cAMP)-dependent protein kinase (protein kinase A).

Therefore:

cAMP stimulates transcription of genes for salivary proteins (eg PRPs)
cAMP stimulates posttranslational modification (eg glycosylation)
cAMP stimulates maturation and translocation of secretory vesicles to the apical membrane
cAMP stimulates exocytosis.

Thus, an increase in the level of cAMP within the cell will stimulate every step involved in protein secretion. Control of protein secretion may therefore be achieved by regulating cAMP levels within the cell. In acinar cells (fig. 2.14), the β-adrenergic receptors which stimulate protein secretion are coupled to G-proteins. Activation of the G-protein G_s by NA binding to acinar cell β-adrenergic receptors stimulates adenylate cyclase to synthesise cAMP from ATP.

cAMP, working through protein kinase A and phosphorylation of target proteins, stimulates every step in the protein biosynthetic and release pathway. Down regulation of the secretory process can be achieved by activation of receptors coupled to an inhibitory G-protein (G_i) which inhibits adenylate cyclase activity.

The four stages in the production of cyclic AMP are illustrated in figure 2.15. First, noradrenaline binds to β-adrenergic receptors(1). The G-protein associated with the receptor moves to an active GTP-bound state(2). Adenylate cyclase is next stimulated by the

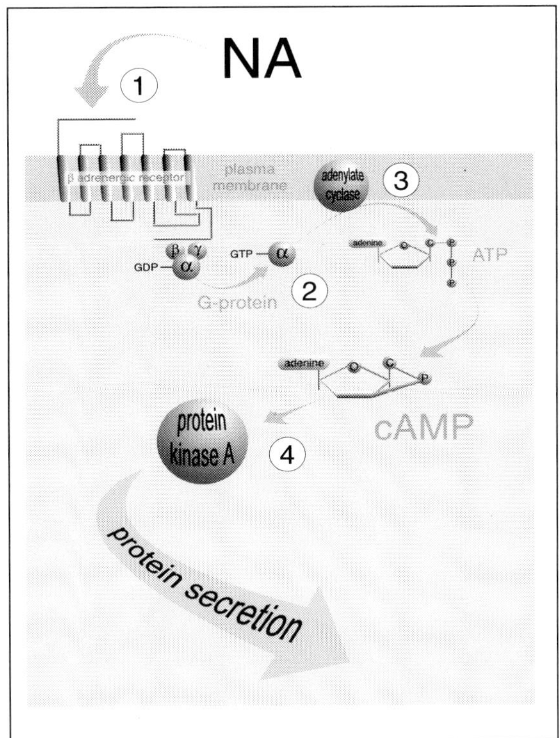

Fig. 2.15 Cyclic AMP production in salivary acinar cells.

G-protein to convert ATP into cAMP(3). Finally cAMP activates protein kinase A which in turn phosphorylates target proteins(4).

There are two types of exocytotic pathways associated with protein secretion in salivary acinar cells. In addition to regulated exocytosis, as described above, there is also the process of constitutive exocytosis.[6] Proteins secreted by this mechanism are not concentrated into secretory vesicles to await exocytotic stimulus; rather there is a continuous flow of protein in small membrane vesicles to the plasma membrane. Any regulation of protein secretion by constitutive exocytosis must occur at the synthetic stage because, once formed, discharge of the protein proceeds automatically without further stimulus.

Activation of adrenergic nerves is not the only way in which protein secretion can be stimulated. In addition to cholinergic and adrenergic neurones, salivary glands also contain peptidergic neurones and acinar cells, in particular mucous acinar cells, have been shown to possess

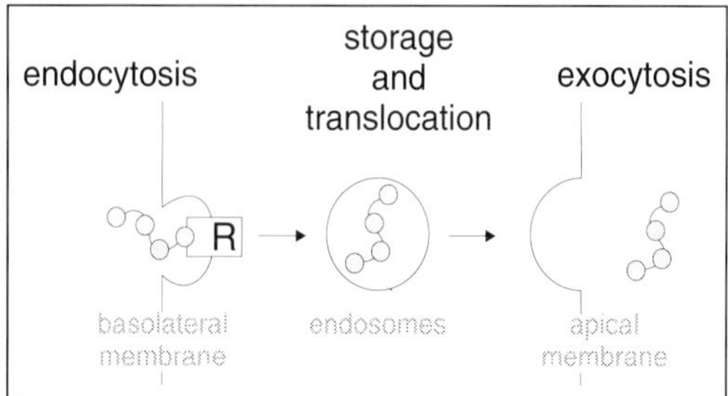

Fig. 2.16 Transepithelial transport of immunoglobulins.

peptide receptors. Vasoactive intestinal polypeptide (VIP), which is present in these peptidergic neurones, stimulates protein secretion, probably via increased cAMP. Peptidergic stimulation also increases blood flow to the salivary glands which may also enhance secretion.

Transepithelial protein transport.

The vast bulk of protein secreted by salivary glands under normal conditions is synthesised within the acinar cells, however there are some plasma proteins found in saliva. Immunoglobulins, such as IgA, which have an important role in the control of oral bacteria (see Chapter 8) are found in saliva; to reach the saliva, from the blood, they must have crossed the epithelial cells. Immunoglobulins cannot cross the plasma membrane, but they may be taken up into cells within membrane vesicles by endocytosis. The basolateral membrane of other transporting epithelia, such as the proximal tubule, the placenta and the small intestine, have been shown to contain a polymeric immunoglobulin receptor which binds immunoglobulins and stimulates endocytosis.

The sequence is outlined in figure 2.16. Firstly there is binding to a receptor at the basolateral membrane and endocytosis. This is followed by transcellular translocation to the apical membrane and then released by exocytosis. The immunoglobulin receptor contains several sorting sequences which direct the immunoglobulin containing vesicles to the golgi apparatus. Such a receptor in salivary acinar cells could be responsible both for the uptake of immunoglobulins from the plasma and for incorporation of immunoglobulins into secretory vesicles so that they may be released along with native proteins following an exocytotic stimulus. Plasma proteins may also reach the saliva via a more pathological paracellular route. The salivary duct epithelium is only a single cell thick, increased intraluminal hydrostatic pressure (which may be produced experimentally by blocking the excretory duct) can force the tight junctions apart and allow, for example, albumin to reach the saliva.

Crosstalk

Although fluid and protein secretion occur by separate mechanisms controlled by different nerves, the separation between the control of protein secretion and fluid and electrolyte secretion breaks down at the second messenger level. Interaction between Ca^{2+} and cAMP mediated events, or crosstalk, allows combination of intracellular signalling pathways into an integrated stimulus-secretion coupling mechanism.

One example of crosstalk may be seen in the regulation of protein kinase activity. Cyclic-AMP-dependent protein kinase is not by any means the only protein kinase in acinar cells. There are many others which may be involved in different aspects of protein synthesis and release; for example, protein kinase C which is stimulated by DAG which in turn is produced along with IP_3 when muscarinic ACh receptors are activated. This is not the only site at which crosstalk can occur, nor is the crosstalk only one way. There is some evidence that Ca^{2+} mobilisation may be modulated by cAMP. Interaction between cyclic-AMP-regulated protein secretion and Ca^{2+} mobilisation also occurs at the final stage of exocytosis because the complex process of docking secretory vesicles to the plasma membrane is dependent on raised intracellular Ca^{2+} concentration.[4]

References

1 Petersen O H. Stimulus-secretion coupling: cytoplasmic calcium signals and the control of ion channels in exocrine acinar cells. *J Physiol* 1992; **448:** 1–51.
2 Berridge M J The biology and medicine of calcium signalling [review]. *Mol Cell Endocrinol* 1994; **98:** 119-124.
3 Smith P M, Gallacher D V. Acetylcholine- and caffeine-evoked repetitive transient Ca^{2+}-activated K^+ and Cl^- currents in mouse submandibular cells. *J Physiol* 1992; **449:** 109-120
4 Thorn P, Lawrie A M, Smith P J, Gallacher D V, Petersen O H. Local and global cytosolic Ca^{2+} oscillations in exocrine cells evoked by agonists and inositol triphosphate. *Cell* 1993; **74:** 661-668.
5 Burgoyne R D, Morgan A. Regulated exocytosis. *Biochem J* 1993; **293:** 305–316.

3

Factors Influencing Salivary Flow Rate and Composition

Colin Dawes

This chapter covers the differences in flow rate and composition between unstimulated saliva (secreted continuously in the absence of exogenous stimulation) and stimulated saliva (secreted usually in response to masticatory or gustatory stimulation), the factors influencing salivary flow rate and composition, and their physiological importance.

Unstimulated saliva

Unstimulated whole saliva is the mixture of secretions which enter the mouth in the absence of exogenous stimuli such as tastants or chewing. It is composed of secretions from the parotid, submandibular, sublingual, and minor mucous glands but it also contains gingival crevicular fluid, desquamated epithelial cells, bacteria, leucocytes (mainly from the gingival crevice), and possibly food residues, blood, and viruses. Unstimulated whole saliva is usually collected with the patient sitting quietly, with the head down and mouth open to allow the saliva to drip from the lower lip into a beaker or similar receptacle over a given time. Alternatively, the patient can spit out the saliva at regular intervals, while swallowing is inhibited. Several large studies of unstimulated salivary flow rates in healthy individuals (Table 3.1) have found the average value for whole saliva to be about 0.3 ml/minute, but the normal range is very large and includes individuals with very low flow rates who do not complain of a dry mouth.

Such a broad normal range makes it difficult to say whether or not a particular individual has an abnormally low flow rate. Unless saliva is almost completely absent, patients can be said to have a dry mouth only on the basis of their subjective symptoms.

Whether the flow rate is high or low is much less important than whether it has changed adversely in a particular individual. Physicians will often take a patient's blood pressure as a yardstick for future

Table 3.1 Unstimulated salivary flow rate (ml/minute) in healthy individuals (Dawes, 1987)

Studies	Type of saliva	Sample number	Mean (ml/minute)	SD*
Andersson *et al.* (1974)	Whole	100	0.39	(0.21)
Becks and Wainwright (1943)	Whole	661	0.32	(0.23)
Heintze *et al.* (1983)	Whole	629	0.31	(0.22)
Shannon and Frome (1973)	Whole	50	0.32	(0.13)
Shannon (1967)	Parotid	4589	0.04	(0.03)
Enfors (1962)	SM**	54	0.10	(0.08)

*Note the very high standard deviation (SD) from the mean, indicating a very wide range of values covering normality.
** SM = Submandibular saliva.

measurements. Dentists, however, do not routinely measure the salivary flow rate, so that when a patient complains of having a dry mouth, it is impossible to judge whether or not a genuine reduction in flow has taken place. It would therefore be very advantageous if dentists included measurement of salivary flow as part of their regular examination.

Just as there are individuals with very little saliva but without discomfort, so there are others with flow rates within the normal range who feel that their mouth is drowning in saliva. This problem is often due to difficulty in swallowing, rather than to a genuinely high flow rate.

Factors affecting the unstimulated salivary flow rate

Many factors influence the unstimulated salivary flow rate (see Table 3.2).

Table 3.2 Factors affecting unstimulated salivary flow rate in healthy subjects

Important factors*	Unimportant factors
Degree of hydration	Gender
Body position	Age (above 15 years)
Exposure to light	Body weight
Previous stimulation	Gland size
Circadian rhythms	Psychic effects
Circannual rhythms	— thought/sight of food
Drugs	— appetite
	— mental stress
	Functional stimulation

* Most factors listed in the first column should be standardised during saliva collection

Degree of hydration

This is potentially the most important factor. When body water content is reduced by 8%, the salivary flow rate decreases to virtually zero. For a person of about 70 kg, comprising about 50 kg of water, 8% dehydration means a loss of 4 litres. In contrast, hyperhydration will increase the salivary flow rate.

Body posture and lighting conditions

Flow rate varies with position and a person when standing or lying will have a higher or lower flow rate, respectively, than when seated. Flow rate also decreases by 30–40% when subjects are blindfolded or in the dark. However, a recent study has shown that salivary flow is not less in blind subjects than in those with normal sight, which suggests that blind individuals eventually adapt to the lack of light entering the eyes.

Biological rhythms

The flow rate of saliva peaks during the late afternoon (the acrophase) and drops to almost zero during sleep (fig. 3.1). It may therefore be important to standardise the time of day at which saliva is collected. This circadian rhythm also has important clinical implications for the timing of oral hygiene. The most important time to clean the teeth is probably at night before going to sleep, since the presence of plaque and food

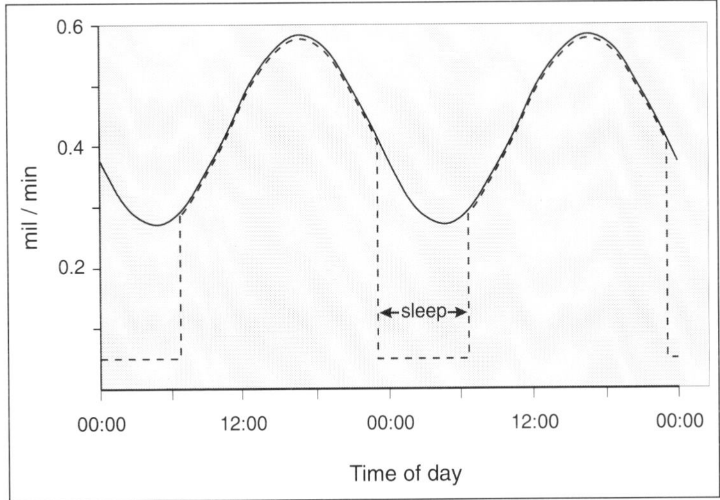

Fig. 3.1 The circadian rhythm in unstimulated salivary flow rate and the idealised effect of sleep (dashed line) from 2300 hours to 0700 hours (from Dawes, 1972).

debris and a greatly reduced salivary flow during sleep provide optimum conditions for dental caries. A study has also shown a circannual rhythm in the flow rate of parotid saliva, with a peak value in the winter. This study, carried out in Texas, found 35% lower flow rates in the summer, and it was assumed that the reduction then was due to dehydration. It would be interesting to repeat the study on subjects living in a temperate climate. Whether this finding means that people are more susceptible to caries in the summer than in the winter would be hard to determine as development of a caries lesion is a long process.

Psychic stimuli

Thinking about food or seeing food are poor stimuli for salivation in humans. It may appear that one salivates at the thought of food, but it is more likely that one merely becomes aware of the pool of saliva present in the floor of the mouth between swallows. Although some researchers have measured a small rise in salivary flow with visual stimuli, others have found no effect. In general, therefore, thinking about or seeing food has little effect in stimulating salivary flow.

Drugs

Many classes of drugs cause a reduction in salivary flow as a side effect (Table 3.3). They may act centrally or directly on the salivary glands (see Chapter 4).

Stimulated saliva

This type of saliva is secreted in response to masticatory or gustatory stimulation, or to other less common stimuli such as activation of the vomiting centre. Several studies of stimulated salivary flow have been done in healthy populations and show a wide variation among individuals (Table 3.4).

Table 3.3 Classes of drugs which may cause xerostomia

Analgesics (narcotics)	Antineoplastics
Anticonvulsants	Antiparasitics
Antinauseants	Appetite suppressants
Anti-Parkinson's agents	Antiemetics
Antipsychotics	Decongestants
Antidepressants	Diuretics
Antihistamines	Expectorants
Antihypertensives	Monoamine oxidase inhibitors
Antispasmodics	Muscle relaxants
Antiarrhythmics	Sedatives/tranquillisers
Anxiolytics	

Table 3.4 Stimulated salivary flow rates in man (Dawes, 1987)

Studies	Type of saliva	Stimulus	Sample number	Mean (ml/min)	SD
Heintze *et al.* (1983)	Whole	Paraffin wax	629	1.6	(2.1)
Shannon and Frome (1973)	Whole	Chewing gum	200	1.7	(0.6)
Shannon *et al.* (1974)	Parotid	Grape candy	368	1.0	(0.5)
Mason *et al.* (1975)	Parotid	Lemon juice	169	1.5	(0.8)
Ericson *et al.* (1972)	Submandibular	1% citric acid	28	0.8	(0.4)

Table 3.5 Factors affecting the flow of stimulated saliva

Nature of stimulus (mechanical, gustatory)	Gag reflex
Vomiting	Olfaction
Smoking	Unilateral stimulation
Gland size	Food intake

The studies used a variety of stimuli, however, and international agreement on a suitable stimulus for experimental use would greatly help comparison of results from different studies.

Factors influencing the stimulated flow rate

Many factors (Table 3.5) influence the stimulated salivary flow rate which, for whole saliva, has an average maximum value of about 7 ml/minute.

Mechanical stimuli

The action of chewing, in the absence of any taste (see results for gum-base in fig. 3.2), will itself stimulate salivation but to a lesser degree than maximum gustatory stimulation with citric acid. Mastication also serves to mix the contents of the mouth, thus increasing the distribution of the different types of saliva around the mouth. Mechanical stimulation of the fauces (the gag reflex) leads to increased salivation.

Vomiting

Salivary flow is increased just prior to and during vomiting. Unfortunately, the increased buffering power of the saliva at the increased flow

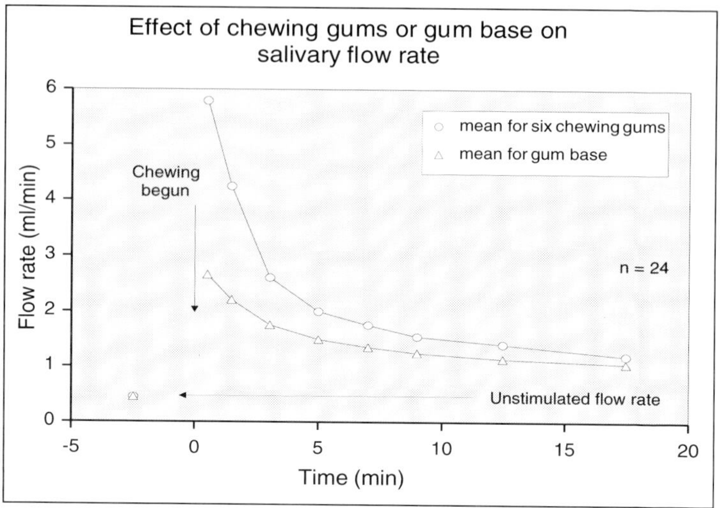

Fig. 3.2 Effect of six chewing gums and gum-base on the flow rate of whole saliva. Unstimulated saliva was collected for 5 minutes prior to chewing gum or gum-base stimulation, which began at time zero.

rate is inadequate to protect the teeth against the erosion caused by the acid gastric juice, particularly in individuals with chronic bulimia.

Gustatory and olfactory stimuli

Acid is the most potent of the four basic taste stimuli, the other three being salt, bitter and sweet. A study done with various concentrations of citric acid found that 5% citric acid stimulated a mean maximum salivary flow rate of about 7 ml/minute. The citric acid was continuously infused into the mouth, and the teeth were covered with a paraffin film to protect them against the acid.

For a clinical evaluation of the residual secretory capacity in patients with xerostomia, a 3% citric acid solution can be applied to the patient's tongue at regular intervals, so that the degree of stimulation is relatively standardised. Alternatively, for research purposes, sour lemon drops (a candy) can be used to standardise the stimulated flow rate from cannulated individual glands. The patient collects saliva into a graduated test tube in front of a mirror. With the aid of a stopwatch, the patients can visualise their salivary flow rate, and adjust it by changing the intensity of sucking on the lemon drop.

Standardisation of flow-rate allows study of the effect of other variables on salivary composition. Olfactory stimuli and tobacco smoking have relatively small effects in stimulating salivary flow.

Unilateral stimulus

If a person habitually chews on one side of the mouth, most of the saliva will be produced by the glands on that side, unless gustatory stimulation is also present.

Gland size

Maximum stimulated flow rate from a single gland is directly related to gland size. The unstimulated flow rate, however, is independent of gland size.

Age

Salivary flow is unrelated to age above 15 years. For a long time it was believed that salivary flow decreased with age, because such studies had been done on institutionalised, medicated patients. More recent research has shown that ageing has little effect on either the unstimulated or stimulated flow rate in normal healthy people who are not on medication. This is surprising because histological studies of salivary glands have shown a reduction in the proportion of secretory cells with age. Presumably there is normally a surplus of secretory tissue. However, many elderly people receive medication and the greater the number of drugs taken, the greater is the tendency for reduction in salivary flow.

Food intake

Surprisingly, very few studies have been carried out with food as the secretory stimulus.

A recent study tested the effects of seven foods. Even the most bland food (boiled rice) elicited 43% of the maximum flow rate produced by 5% citric acid. Rhubarb pie, which is both acidic and sweet, elicited 70% of the maximum flow rate. Further study showed that it was the gustatory stimulus provided by the food, rather than the mechanical stimulus of chewing, which was mainly responsible for these relatively high flow rates.

With chewing gum (fig. 3.2), the flow rate is high initially but after about ten minutes, as the flavour and sweetness leach out and only the gum-base remains, it falls to the rate obtained by chewing gum base alone, namely to two to three times the unstimulated rate. However, since gum is usually chewed for a long time (20–30 minutes), even this increase in salivary flow over a prolonged period may be beneficial to those with a dry mouth.

Salivary flow rate and oral health

The unstimulated flow rate is more important than the stimulated flow for oral comfort, since only a small fraction of the day is spent eating. However, stimulation of the glands through mastication is beneficial in terms of promoting clearance of food from the mouth (see Chapter 5) and may help by causing an increase in the unstimulated flow rate. Unfortunately, little can be done to influence the unstimulated flow rate on a long term basis, but a recent study has shown that chewing gum (sugar free), used by students over a long period of time, produced a small rise in the unstimulated, but not stimulated, flow rate. This result suggests that if the glands are stimulated, their activity may increase.

Carbohydrate clearance from the oral cavity

One major effect of saliva is the clearance of carbohydrate from the mouth (see Chapter 5). The more rapid the flow, the faster the carbohydrate is cleared. This is true whether the saliva is unstimulated or stimulated, for example by chewing gum. If the gum contains sweeteners such as xylitol or sorbitol, then the increased salivary flow will be very effective in carbohydrate clearance.

Total daily salivary flow

If the average unstimulated flow rate over a waking period of 16 hours is about 0.3 ml/minute, the total volume will be about 300 ml of saliva. During sleep, the maximum flow will fall to less than 0.1 ml/minute, producing less than 40 ml of saliva in 7 hours. The average time spent eating each day has been estimated as 54 minutes. Studies with various foods suggested that during eating the average stimulated flow rate is about 4 ml/minute. So about 200 ml of saliva per day will be produced during meals. Thus the total daily flow of saliva amounts to about 500–600 ml/24 hours, which is much less than the 1500 ml/24 hours quoted in many textbooks.

The composition of saliva

The composition of saliva is affected by a number of factors (Table 3.6), such as the type of salivary gland producing the saliva. For example, most of the amylase in saliva is produced by the parotid glands while blood-group substances are derived mainly from the minor mucous glands.

Contribution of different glands

The parotid glands normally contribute about 20% of the total volume of unstimulated saliva, while the submandibular glands contribute 65%, the sublingual 7–8%, and the minor mucous glands 7–8%. At high flow rates, the parotid becomes the dominant gland, contributing about 50% of the whole saliva.

Flow Rate

The main factor affecting the composition of saliva is the flow rate (fig. 3.3). As the flow rate increases, the pH and concentrations of some constituents rise (for example, protein, sodium, chloride, bicarbonate), while those of others fall (for example, magnesium and phosphate). The fluoride concentration in saliva is about 1 µmol/l and is relatively independent of flow rate but with a slight increase at low unstimulated flow rates.

Duration of stimulation

If the salivary flow rate is held constant, then the composition of the saliva depends on the duration of stimulation. So, saliva collected at a constant flow rate for 2 minutes will have a different composition from saliva collected at the same flow rate for 10–15 minutes. For instance, the bicarbonate concentration increases with duration of stimulation, whereas the chloride level falls in a reciprocal manner. The salivary composition will vary depending on whether the gland has been stimulated during the previous hour.

Nature of the stimulus

Different stimuli have an effect on salivary composition, mainly because of their effect on the rate of flow. When the four basic taste stimuli (salt, acid, bitter, and sweet) were tested under constant flow conditions,

Table 3.6 Factors affecting salivary composition

Species	Hormones
Glandular source	Pregnancy
Flow rate	Genetic polymorphism
Duration of stimulation	Antigenic stimulus
Previous stimulation	Exercise
Biological rhythms	Drugs
Nature of stimulus	Various diseases
Plasma composition (diet)	

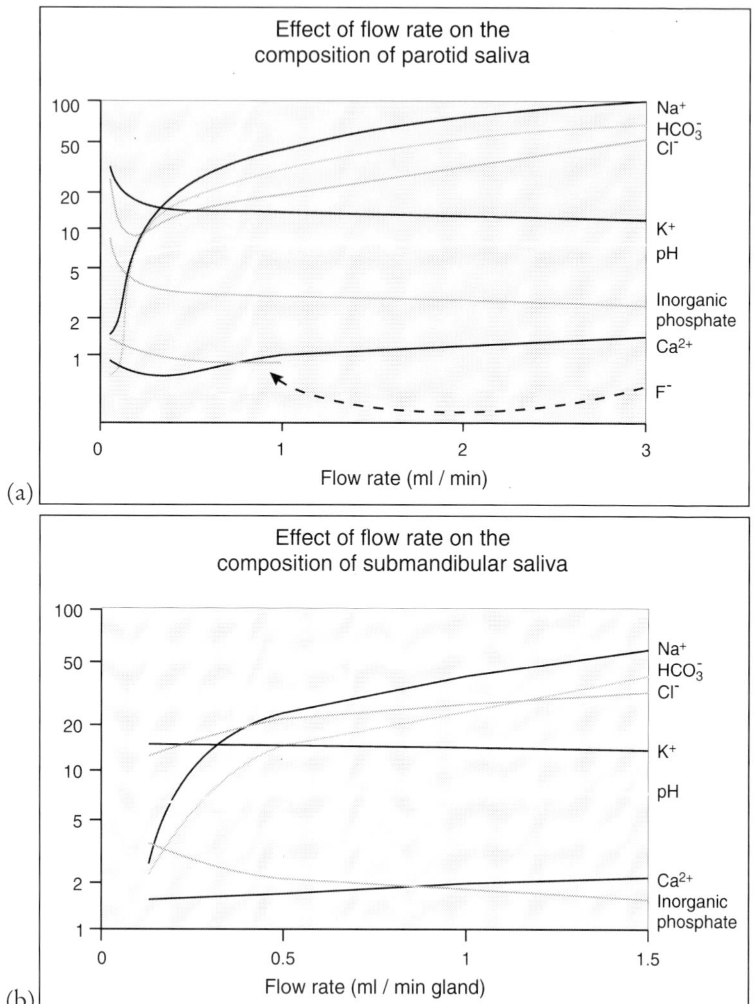

Fig. 3. 3 The effects of flow rate and duration of stimulation on the concentrations (mmol/l except for F, which is µmol/l) of some components of (a) parotid saliva and (b) submandibular saliva.

the type of stimulus used had virtually no effect on the electrolyte composition of parotid saliva, but the taste of salt stimulated much the highest protein content. There does not seem to be any physiological reason why this should be so. The increase occurred with all protein components; different stimuli did not elicit secretion of different proteins. Acid is the most potent stimulus for salivary secretion and leads to production of an alkaline saliva. At one time it was thought that this was a beneficial adaptation to the nature of the stimulus. However, it is now known that the pH of saliva is dependent mainly on the flow rate and is independent of the nature of the stimulus.

Circadian rhythms

As with flow rate, salivary composition shows rhythms of high amplitude. For instance, sodium and chloride levels peak in the early morning, while the rhythm in potassium concentration is 12 hours out of phase. The peak protein concentration is in the late afternoon.

Saliva and taste

When saliva is first secreted by the acinar cells of the salivary glands, its electrolyte composition resembles that of an ultrafiltrate of plasma. As the saliva passes down the salivary duct, the gland expends energy to re-absorb virtually all the sodium chloride and most of the bicarbonate, while secreting potassium (fig. 3.4). By the time the salivary secretion reaches the opening of the main excretory duct into the mouth its osmotic pressure is only about one sixth of those in plasma and in the acinar cells.

Why does the salivary gland go to so much trouble to produce a hypotonic saliva? The probable reason is to facilitate taste. Taste buds rapidly adapt to the taste of any solution in the mouth including, of course, saliva. Thus, if saliva had the same salt concentration as plasma

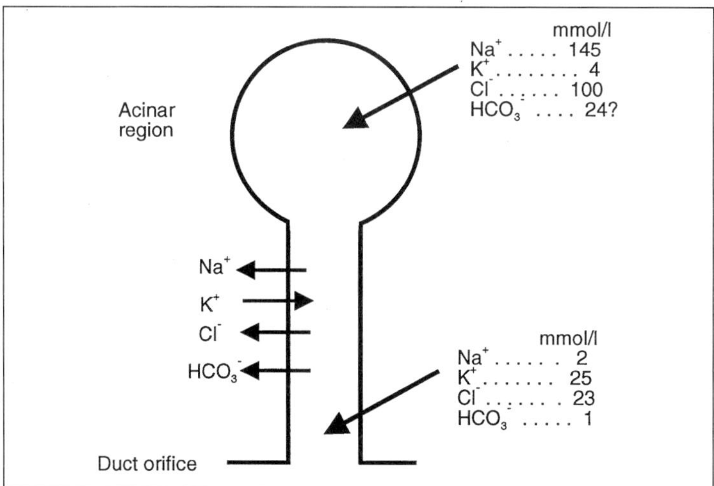

Fig. 3.4 Changes in some electrolyte concentrations as unstimulated parotid saliva moves down the salivary duct.

Table 3.7 Relation of plasma and saliva compositions* to taste thresholds

	Salt		Sour		Sweet	Bitter
	Na^+	Cl^-	H^+	HCO_3^-	Glucose	Urea
Plasma	145	101	4×10^{-5}	24	4.5	6
Saliva	4	16	4×10^{-4}	3	0.05	5
	NaCl		HCl	$NaHCO_3$	Sucrose	Urea
Taste recognition threshold	12		0.8	10	30	90

*All concentrations are in mmol/l.

(which is very high), we would be unable to taste salt concentrations lower than that in plasma. Hence the reabsorption of sodium and chloride during saliva production, and the resultant hypotonicity of saliva, facilitate our ability to taste salt.

Unstimulated saliva is particularly well adapted to facilitate the sensation of taste. Besides being low in sodium chloride (salt), it is also low in glucose (sweet), buffering capacity (acid), and urea (bitter). Taste recognition thresholds are compared with concentration levels in plasma and in unstimulated saliva in Table 3.7.

The buffering ability of saliva

Proteins

The concentration of protein in saliva is only about one-thirtieth of that in plasma, so that too few amino acids are present to have a significant buffering effect at the usual pH of the oral cavity.

Phosphate

As with proteins, there is too little phosphate in saliva to act as a significant buffer.

Bicarbonate

This is the most important buffering system in saliva but only at high flow rates, when it is an important buffer against acid produced by dental plaque. Its concentration varies from less than 1 mmol/l in unstimulated parotid saliva to almost 60 mmol/l at very high flow rates, with whole saliva elicited by chewing gum having a bicarbonate concentration of about 15 mmol/l. Thus, in unstimulated saliva, the level of bicarbonate ions is too low to be an effective buffer. This allows us to taste acid put into the mouth, since the resulting fall in pH can stimulate gustatory receptors.

Table 3.8 Calcium and inorganic phosphate concentrations in saliva

	Plasma	Parotid saliva	SM* saliva	MMG** secretions
Calcium (mmol/l)	2.5	0.9	2.0	2.1
Phosphate (mmol/l)	1.0	3.5	2.9	0.4
Flow rate***	-	1.2	1.2	-

*SM = submandibular saliva; **MMG = minor mucous gland; ***ml/minute/gland pair

pH

Salivary pH is dependent on the bicarbonate concentration, an increase in which results in an increase in pH. The relationship between the pH and the bicarbonate concentration is given by the Henderson-Hasselbalch equation, $pH = pK + \log[HCO_3^-]/[H_2CO_3]$, in which the pK (about 6.1) and $[H_2CO_3^-]$ (about 1.2 mmol/l) are virtually independent of the flow rate.

At very low flow rates, the pH can be as low as 5.3, rising to 7.8 at very high parotid flow rates. Individuals with xerostomia will thus have a low salivary pH and a low salivary buffering capacity because of the low bicarbonate concentration (fig. 3.3).

Calcium and phosphate concentrations

Calcium and phosphate (PO_4^{3-}) ions, along with hydroxyl ions, maintain the saturation of saliva with respect to tooth mineral, and are therefore important in calculus formation and in protecting against the development of caries. Saliva contains less calcium but more phosphate than does plasma (Table 3.8). The mechanisms responsible for a higher concentration of phosphate in saliva than in plasma are uncertain. In addition, secretions from different salivary glands have different concentrations of calcium and phosphate. For example, parotid saliva contains less calcium but more inorganic phosphate than does submandibular saliva, while the minor mucous gland secretions are very low in phosphate (Table 3.8).

A decreasing phosphate concentration at high flow rates (fig. 3.3) would seem to be bad for teeth, as it might result in undersaturation of the saliva with respect to tooth mineral. However, as the flow rate increases, so does the bicarbonate concentration and therefore the pH of saliva. A high pH alters the proportions of the four different phosphate species (H_3PO_4, $H_2PO_4^-$, HPO_4^{2-}, and PO_4^{3-}) such that there is a fall in $H_2PO_4^-$ and a slight increase in HPO_4^{2}, but a dramatic increase in PO_4^{3-}. It is the PO_4^{3-} which is the important ionic species with respect to the solubility of tooth mineral (see Chapter 9). Thus, although the total level of phosphate falls with increasing flow rate, the concentration of PO_4^{3-} actually increases (fig. 3.5) as much as 40-fold when flow rate increases from the unstimulated level to high flow rates. If, therefore, we consider the components of the ion product determining the solubility of tooth mineral, all three (Ca^{2+}, PO_4^{3-}, OH^-) increase with salivary flow. Thus the higher the flow rate, the more effective is saliva in reducing demineralisation and promoting remineralisation of the teeth. This also means, however, that the higher the flow rate, the greater the potential for calculus formation to occur.

Minor mucous gland secretions

These differ in several ways from the secretions of the major glands (submandibular, sublingual, and parotid). They are extremely viscous, very low in phosphate, they contain virtually no bicarbonate, so they are very poorly buffered, the main ions are sodium, potassium, and chloride, and they are the main source of secretory IgA in the mouth. It is unfortunate that, mainly because of collection difficulties, these secretions have received little study despite their being in intimate contact with most of the oral mucosa and hard tissues.

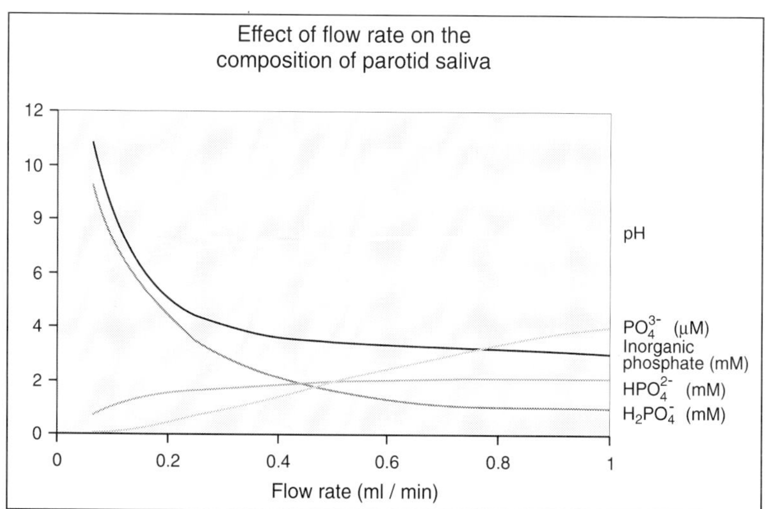

Fig. 3.5 The effect of salivary flow rate on the concentrations of the different species of inorganic phosphate in parotid saliva. Note that the PO_4^{3-} concentration is in μmol/l, whereas the concentrations of the other species are in mmol/l.

Summary — Clinical Highlights

Salivary flow rate is nearly zero in sleep. Maximum cariogenic activity is likely to occur when people eat carbohydrate at night and then do not brush their teeth before going to sleep.

Dentists should be aware that many patients are taking medications (for example beta blockers) that have a tendency to reduce salivary flow, making the patient more susceptible to dental caries.

When salivary flow rate increases, this results in a higher salivary pH and bicarbonate content, which have beneficial effects on plaque pH if the stimulus to salivation does not include acid or additional sugar. The increased flow rate will itself tend to remove carbohydrate from the mouth, and stir up the very thin film of saliva (see Chapter 5) which covers the oral surfaces. The bicarbonate will tend to diffuse into plaque and act as a buffer by neutralising acids present in the plaque, and increase the time for remineralisation of early caries.

Dentists should measure the unstimulated salivary flow rate of patients at appropriate intervals, as this would provide baseline values for future comparison. A very low salivary flow rate is an indication of caries susceptibility and influences the preventive treatment provided by the dentist.

Further reading

1 Dawes C. Saliva and dental caries. *In* Nikiforuk G, ed. *Understanding dental caries.* 1 Etiology and mechanisms. Basic clinical aspects. Volume 1, pp 236–260. Basel: Karger, 1985.

2 Dawes C. Physiological factors affecting salivary flow rate, oral sugar clearance, and the sensation of dry mouth in man. *J Dent Res* 1987; **66:** 648 653.

3 Mandel I D. The role of saliva in maintaining oral homeostasis. *J Am Dent Assoc* 1989; **119:** 298–304.

4 Tenovuo J, Lagerlöf F. Saliva. In: Thylstrup A, Fejerskov O, eds. T*extbook of clinical cariology.* 2nd ed. pp 17–43. Copenhagen: Munksgaard, 1994.

5 Watanabe S, Dawes C. The effects of different foods and concentrations of citric acid on the flow rate of whole saliva in man. *Arch Oral Biol* 1988; **33:** 1–5.

4

Xerostomia: diagnosis, management and clinical complications

Leo M Sreebny

'How dry I am,
How dry I am,
Nobody cares,
Nobody knows'

(Lyrics from an old American 'Prohibition' refrain)

Fluids of the body, like blood, urine and even sweat and tears, have been widely used as indicators of health and disease. Only one has been virtually ignored — saliva. Yet, this shunned and rejected secretion, protects the teeth and soft oral tissues, aids in the selection and preparation of food for digestion and assists with speech. Moreover, it is a sensitive indicator of serious systemic diseases and conditions.

Xerostomia (dry mouth) is the subjective feeling of oral dryness. It is generally accompanied by salivary gland hypofunction (SGH) and a severe reduction in the secretion of unstimulated (resting) whole saliva.

The flow rate of whole saliva

As given in Chapter 3, the normal rate of flow (fig. 4.1) of unstimulated whole saliva (UFR) is approximately 0.3 ml/min; that of stimulated whole saliva (SFR) about 1–2 ml/min. When the UFR falls to about 50% of its normal value, subjects complain of oral dryness.[1] Thus, for a person with a UFR of 0.30 ml/min, dryness would be noted if the UFR fell to 0.15 ml/min. In the unstimulated state the two parotid glands contribute about 30% of the whole saliva; the combined submandibular/ sublingual glands, about 70%. It can be shown that for a reduction of 50% of the UFR (ie when xerostomia is perceived), more than one gland must be affected (Table 4.1). Thus xerostomia is caused by multi-glandular (ie probably systemic) disease.

Materials: Collecting vessel (Sialometer, ProFlow Inc., Amityville, New York; or graduated test-tube (volume ~12 ml; divisions = 0.1 ml, obtainable from chemical supply houses); stop-watch; paraffin wax (Orion Diagnostica, Espoo, Finland); 2% citric acid (prepared by a pharmacist).

General Information: Saliva is collected after an overnight fast or at least 1.5 hours after eating. Patients are instructed not to put anything in their mouth before coming in for the test. The collection procedure should be performed in a quiet area.

The Collection of Unstimulated Whole Saliva: Patients are advised that a very small amount of saliva will ooze into their mouth in the unstimulated state and that the objective of the test is to measure the rate of flow of this secretion. Therefore, they should not swallow during this procedure. They are told to sit still, bow their head and try not to move during the test. Immediately before the test begins they should swallow any residual saliva that may be in their mouth. The saliva is allowed to accumulate for 2 minutes and then expectorated into the collecting vessel. If insufficient saliva is obtained, the test may be conducted for a longer period of time; often for 5 minutes. The physical characteristics of the saliva are noted and the volume is recorded. Flow is expressed as ml/min.

The Collection of Stimulated Whole Saliva: A standard piece of paraffin wax (1.5 g; melting point = 42°C) is used. The patient is asked to chew the wax, without swallowing, and expectorate the stimulated saliva into the collecting vessel. Two, or if needed, 5 minute samples are collected. As with the unstimulated saliva, the physical characteristics of the saliva and the volume are recorded and the flow is expressed as ml/min.

A 2% citric acid solution may be employed to stimulate saliva in edentulous patients or in those who cannot chew the wax. The dorso-lateral part of the tongue may be swabbed every 30 seconds for a period of 2 minutes. The saliva is then collected after 2 to 5 minutes.

Normal Reference Values: The unstimulated flow rate generally varies between 0.3 and 0.4 ml/min. Values < 0.1 ml should be considered abnormal. The normal stimulated flow rate varies between 1 to 2 ml/min. Values < 0.5 ml/min should be viewed as abnormal.

Fig. 4.1 Determination of the flow rate of whole saliva

Table 4.1 Projected flow of whole saliva minus the contributions of select salivary glands

Salivary gland profile	Flow rate (ml/ min)
Mean, unstimulated flow rate (UFR), whole saliva	0.30
Xerostomia perceived at ~50% of UFR	*0.15**
UFR minus the contribution of 1 parotid gland	0.25
UFR minus the contribution of 2 parotid glands	0.20
UFR minus the contribution of 1 pair of SM/SL glands	0.20
UFR minus the contribution of 2 pairs of SM/SL glands	*0.10*
UFR minus the contribution of 1 parotid and 1 pair of SM/SL glands	*0.15*
UFR minus the contribution of 2 parotids and 1 pair of SM/SL glands	*0.10*
UFR minus the contribution of 1 parotid and 2 pairs of SM/SL glands	*0.05*

**Italic* type indicates presence of xerostomia

Since flow rate varies widely among individuals (see Chapter 3), so too will the point at which they complain of dry mouth. Dentists and physicians rarely measure the flow rates of saliva in their patients so the 'cut-off' point for a specific patient is rarely known. In general, subjects whose UFR is ≤ 0.1 ml/min or whose SFR is ≤ 0.5 ml/min should be viewed with concern. However, these values should be used in a rigid manner. Low flow rates, in the absence of any symptoms or clinical signs associated with xerostomia, may not indicate the presence of disease. Conversely, subjects may complain of oral dryness at higher flow rates. Since saliva plays such an important role in the health of oral tissues, it is prudent to suggest that dentists should obtain baseline UFRs and SFRs of whole saliva on all of their patients.

The causes of salivary gland hypofunction and xerostomia

Saliva is produced by the salivary glands. These glands may be viewed as a huge factory which, under normal circumstances, imports raw materials and manufactures a 'soft drink' with the aid of complex, electrically driven machinery. Any reduction in the availability of the raw materials, damage to the machinery or an interruption of the electricity will halt or impair production. Translating this analogy to the salivary glands, any interference with the supply of metabolites, including water, damage to the glands or failure in neural transmission can induce a reduction in the synthesis of saliva. The conditions which can induce salivary hypofunction follow (Table 4.2). Implicit in this list is

Table 4.2 The causes of salivary gland hypofunction and xerostomia

1. Water/metabolite loss
Dehydration:
Impaired water intake
Loss of water through the skin (fever, burns, excessive sweating)
Blood loss
Emesis
Diarrhoea
Renal water loss:
polyuria (Diabetes Insipidus)
osmotic diuresis (Diabetes Mellitus)
Protein calorie malnutrition
2. Damage to the salivary glands
Therapeutic irradiation to the head and neck region
Autoimmune diseases (Sjögren's syndrome [SS], graft-versus-host-disease [GHVD], systemic lupus erythematosis [SLE], rheumatoid arthritis [RA], etc.)
HIV-1 infection (HIV disease)
Ageing (?)
3. Interference with neural transmission
Medications/drugs
Autonomic dysfunction (eg ganglionic neuropathy)
Conditions affecting the CNS (eg Alzheimer's disease)
Psychogenic disorders (depression, anxiety)
Trauma
Decrease in mastication

the fact that xerostomia is caused by systemic diseases or conditions. Indeed, with the possible exception of mouth breathing (evaporation), local factors, *per se*, do not induce oral dryness. Several conditions are of particular import.

Drugs

A common cause of SGH and xerostomia is the use of xerogenic drugs. Hundreds of prescription and over-the-counter medications have the capacity to induce oral dryness. The more drugs one consumes, the greater the prevalence of xerostomia (fig. 4.2). In general, the desiccation due to drugs is reversible. Elimination of the medications that induce the xerostomia restores the flow to normal or near-normal rates. A listing of select xerogenic drugs is shown in Table 4.3 (page 48).

Therapeutic irradiation

Xerostomia, SGH, mucositis and dysphagia are commonly seen in patients whose salivary glands have been irradiated for oral and facial

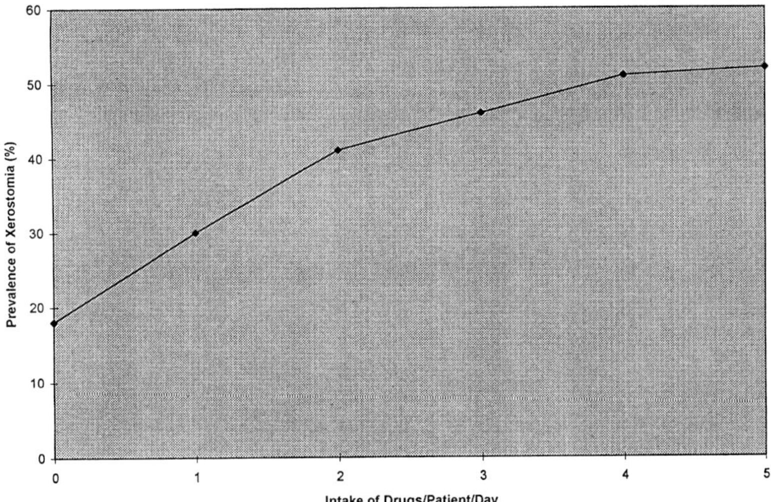

Fig. 4.2 The relationship between drugs and dry mouth.

cancer. The sensation of oral dryness occurs early in the course of radiation. It has been shown that 24 hours after the administration of only 225 rads, there is already a 50% decrease in the resting flow of parotid saliva.[2] With greater amounts of radiation, this deficit increases to over 90%.

Systemic diseases and conditions

Xerostomia is associated with a number of systemic diseases (Table 4.2). One disease in which desiccation plays a particularly prominent role is Sjögren's syndrome (SS), a chronic, multisystem, autoimmune disorder. It is characterised by 1. generalised exocrine gland dysfunction, 2. serologic abnormalities and 3. organ system changes. There are two forms: a primary (Sicca) form, characterised by xerostomia and keratoconjuctivitis sicca (dry eyes); and a secondary form, in which one or both of these symptoms is accompanied by an autoimmune disease, usually rheumatoid arthritis. Other autoimmune disorders which may be associated with it are systemic lupus erythematosus (SLE) and scleroderma (progressive systemic sclerosis, PSS). After rheumatoid arthritis, SS is the most common rheumatoid disease. The syndrome is more common in women (9:1) and it is most often observed in patients over 40 years of age. Xerostomia is observed in over 90% of the patients. The principal histopathologic finding in the salivary glands, especially the parotid, is a lymphoepithelial lesion.

Table 4.3 Select xerogenic medications (classes and generic names)

Analgesics
- *Non-narcotics: NSAIDs*
  - Ibuprofen
  - Fenoprofen
  - Etodolac
  - Nabumetone
- *Narcotics*
  - Morphine sulphate
  - Hydromorphone HCl
  - Oxymorphone
  - Hydrocodone
  - Levorphanol tartrate
  - Methadone HCl
  - Meperedine
  - Fentanyl
  - Sufentanil
  - Codeine phosphate
  - Oxycodone
  - Propoxyphene

Appetite suppressants
- *Amphetamines*
  - Benzphetamine
  - Biphetamine
  - Dextroamphetamine
  - Methamphetamine
- *Non-amphetamines*
  - Phentermine
  - Phendimetrazine tartrate
  - Fenfluramine

Anti-acne preparation
- Isotretinoin

Anti-arthritic
- Piroxicam

Anti-cholinergics and anti-spasmodics (urinary)
- Flavoxate HCl
- Oxybutynin HCl

Anti-cholinergics and anti-spasmodics (GI tract)
- *Anti-cholinergics*
  - Atropine
  - Scopolamine
  - L-hyoscyamine
  - Belladonna alkaloids
- *Quartenary anti-cholinergics*
  - Methscopolamine
  - Clidinium bromide
  - Glycopyrrolate
  - Oxyphenonium bromide
  - Propantheline bromide
  - Tridihexethyl chloride
- *Anti-spasmodics*
  - Dicyclomine HCl

Anti-diarrhoeals
- Diphenoxylate HCl with atropine sulphate
- Loperamide

Anti-emetics
- Benzquinamide HCl
- Diphenidol

Anti-histamines
- *Ethanolamines*
  - Diphenhydramine HCl
  - Clemastine
- *Ethylenediamines*
  - Chlorpheniramine maleate
  - Bromphemiramine maleate
  - Triprolidine
- *Phenothiazines*
  - Promethazine
  - Trimeprazine
- *Piperidines*
  - Cyproheptidine
  - Azatadine
  - Phenindamine

Anti-hypertensives
- *ACE inhibitors*
  - Captopril
  - Enalapril
  - Fosinopril
  - Lisinopril
  - Quinapril HCl
  - Ramipril
- *Anti-adrenergic agents (centrally acting)*
  - Methyldopa
  - Clonidine HCl
  - Guanabenz
- *Anti-adrenergic agents (peripherally acting)*
  - Reserpine
  - Guanethidine
  - Guanadrel
  - Prazosin
- *Anti-adrenergic agents (beta-adrenergic blockers)*
  - Metoprolol
  - Atenolol
  - Nadolol
  - Pindolol
  - Propanolol
- *Calcium channel blocking agents*
  - Nifedipine

Diltiazem HCl
Verapamil
Anti-hypertensives + diuretics (examples)
Clonidine HCl + chlorthalidone
Nadolol + bendroflumethazide
Propanolol HCl + hydrochlorothiazide
Anti-Parkinson drugs
Benztropine mesylate MSD
Biperiden HCl and Biperiden lactate
Bromocriptine mesylate
Carbidopa/Levidopa
Diphenhydramine HCl
Hyoscyamine sulphate
Procyclidine HCl
Trihexphenidyl HCl
Diuretics
Thiazides (oral dryness and thirst are signs of electrolyte imbalance)
Chlorothiazide
Hydrochlorothiazide
Bendroflumethiazide
Cyclothiazide
Methyclothiazide
Benzthiazide
Hydroflumethiazide
Trichlormethiazide
Polythiazide
Quinethazone
Metolazone
Chlorthalidone
Indapamide
Flumethiazide
Loop diuretics (oral dryness/thirst are signs of electrolyte imbalance)
Furosemide
Ethacrynic acid
Bumetanide
Psychotropic agents
Anti-anxiety agents
Benzodiazepines
Oxazepam
Lorazepam
Alprazolam
Diazepam
Halazepam
Prazepam
Chlorazepate dipotassium
Anti-depressants
MAO inhibitors
Phenelzine sulphate
Tranylcypromine sulphate
Serotonin uptake inhibitors
Venlafaxine HCl
Paroxetine HCl
Fluoxetine HCl
Sertraline HCl
Tetracyclics
Maprotiline HCl
Tricyclics
Tertiary amines
Amitriptyline
Imipramine
Doxepin
Trimipramine
Secondary amines
Amoxapine
Nortriptyline
Desipramine
Protriptyline
Tetracyclic
Maprotiline
Miscellaneous
Trazadone
Anti-psychotic agents
Phenothiazines
Aliphatic
Chlorpromazine
Promazine
Piperidine
Mesoridazine
Thoridiazine
Piperazine
Perphenazine
Prochlorperazine
Fluphenazine
Trifluoperazine
Thioxanthenes
Chlorprothixene
Thiothixene
Butyrophenone
Haloperidol
Dihydroindolone
Molindone
Dibenzoazepine
Loxapine
Diphenylbutyl piperidine
Pimozide
Anti-manic agents
Lithium

In its mature form, this lesion is characterised by 1. lymphoreticular cell proliferation, 2. ductal hyperplasia and metaplasia and 3. acinar cell degeneration and atrophy. These histologic changes may also be observed in biopsies of the minor salivary glands of the lip and palate.

Ageing

It is widely believed that we 'dry up' as we get older. Post mortem studies have demonstrated that, with age, the parenchyma of the salivary glands are gradually replaced by fat, connective tissue and oncocytes. But functional studies, in the living, indicate that ageing *per se* does not lead to a diminution in the capacity of these glands to produce saliva. Since most organs are able to compensate for modest losses of tissue, this is not surprising. Several studies have shown that in healthy, unmedicated individuals there is no decrease in the flow of whole or parotid saliva with age; one of these was a 10-year, longitudinal study.[3,4] It appears, however, that there may be a progressive, though minor, loss in the flow of saliva from the submandibular glands.[5] As stated earlier, dryness is observed when there is a 50% decrease in the function of the salivary glands. It is doubtful whether the changes observed in ageing are of this order of magnitude.

Older people, however, consume more medications and suffer from more diseases than younger people. It is likely that the dryness frequently observed in aged individuals is due to these facts, rather than to the ageing process.

Decreased mastication

Decreased mastication induces salivary gland atrophy and an accompanying decrease in the synthesis and secretion of saliva.[6–9] These data strongly suggest that the partial or total loss of teeth, the presence of temporomandibular dysfunction, extensive caries, periodontal disease, pain and other clinical conditions may contribute to the onset of oral dryness and SGH. So too will the consumption of soft foods or liquid diets. Implicit in these findings is that dentists should place a high priority on the restoration of the oral cavity to maximal function.

The epidemiology of xerostomia

Studies conducted on outpatients or in the general population have shown that about one out of four patients complain of xerostomia or symptoms associated with it.[10–12] About 40% of the elderly complain of dry mouth.[13–16] Thus, contrary to what is generally believed,[11] dry mouth is a common condition.

The clinical signs associated with xerostomia

Xerostomia is rarely a solitary symptom. When present for extended periods of time it induces a wide variety of other oral symptoms. In addition, patients with dry mouth frequently complain of generalised desiccation. The symptoms usually associated with xerostomia are shown in Table 4.4.

The oral signs associated with xerostomia and SGH are primarily the result of a reduction in the protective functions of saliva. Both the hard and the soft oral tissues are affected. Patients with dry mouth often demonstrate signs of extensive dental decay. In patients who receive regular dental care, the presence of a large numbers of fillings indicates a past history of active caries. The mouths of those who are not the beneficiaries of regular dental care often display signs of active, sometimes rampant, caries. Moreover, the carious lesions are often located at sites which normally do not show signs of decay. Included among these are the lower anterior teeth, the cusps and cervical regions of the teeth, and surfaces of teeth which were recently restored.

An important, but generally neglected, feature of SGH is the decrease in oral clearance. Under normal conditions, the oral cavity

Table 4.4 Symptoms frequently associated with xerostomia

Oral	Systemic
Saliva: decrease in amount, foamy, viscous, ropy (increase in 'spinnbarkeit')	*Throat*: dryness, hoarseness, persistent dry cough
Lips: dry, cracked, fissured (cheilosis)	*Nose*: dryness, frequent crust formation, decrease in olfactory acuity
Tongue: burning (glossopyrosis), pain (glossodynia)	*Eyes*: dryness, burning, itching, gritty sensation, feeling that the lids stick together, blurred vision, sensitivity to light
Cheeks: dry	*Skin*: dryness, butterfly rash, vasculitis
Salivary glands: Swelling, pain	*Joints*: arthritis; pain, swelling, stiffness
Thirst: frequent ingestion of fluids, especially while eating; keep water at bedside	*GI tract*: constipation
Mastication: difficulty with eating dry foods; difficulty with the use of a denture	*Vagina*: dryness, burning, itching, history of recurrent fungal infections, dyspareunia
Swallowing: difficulty with (dysphagia)	*General symptoms*: fatigue, weakness, generalised aching, weight loss, depression
Speech: difficulty with (dysphonia)	
Taste: difficulty with (dysgeusia)	

readily 'clears' or eliminates substances present in it. The principal mechanism involved in clearance is swallowing. Over 90% of substances contained in saliva eg foods, sugar and bacteria, are effectively eliminated from the mouth by the initial swallowing reflex. The remainder is usually eliminated after about 30 minutes. So effective is this mechanism, it is difficult, in the healthy individual, to establish foreign organisms in the mouth. In xerostomia, however, the decrease in the volume of saliva and the presence of dysphagia, creates a situation wherein substances tend to remain in the oral cavity for long periods of time. Indeed, it has recently been shown that a 0.12% solution of chlorhexidine is retained in the mouth for up to 4 hours following a rinse in xerostomic patients. The depression of clearance has important consequences. The retention of sugars, for example, enhances the onset of dental caries; the retention of Gram negative bacilli, induces a particularly virulent form of pneumonia in the elderly.

Candidiasis is another common finding in patients with xerostomia. It often affects the tongue and the lips or it may be present on the palate, underneath a denture. The candidiasis may appear as a deep red, erythematous lesion; as a white to ecru removable plaque; as a white tan pseudomembrane; or, as cheilosis, a fissure or crack at the corners of the mouth.

The buccal mucosa may appear pale and feel dry. The tongue may demonstrate signs of lobulation or fissuring. A tongue-blade, placed on the dorsum of the tongue, will tend to stick to it. On occasion, the patient may demonstrate bilateral or unilateral swelling of the parotid or submandibular salivary glands. Often, it is not possible to 'milk' any saliva from the orifices of Stenson's or Wharton's ducts. Sometimes, the secretions obtained from these ducts are thicker than normal, do not flow as freely as normal saliva, and tend to adhere, as a 'drop', at the duct orifice.[17]

A number of non-oral clinical signs are associated with xerostomia. These are a reflection of the generalised exocrinopathy which is present in this condition. Eye changes include keratoconjunctivitis sicca and decreased lacrimation. Nasal dryness is present and it may be accompanied by nasal crusts, epistaxes and a decrease in olfactory acuity. Diminished sweat gland activity leads to xeroderma. And a decrease in the production of mucous by cells which line the respiratory tract may lead to recurrent bronchitis, pneumonitis and interstitial fibrosis. Moreover, the decrease in the production of saliva, as well as in the mucins which coat the gastrointestinal tract, may lead to pharyngitis, laryngitis, reflux oesophagitis, heartburn and constipation. Vaginal dryness and the accompanying decrease in the flow of vaginal secretions may lead to recurrent fungal infections. Severe, repeated episodes of vaginal dryness may lead to dyspareunia.[18,19] Many of these signs are observed in patients with Sjögren's syndrome.

Salivary function tests

Salivary function tests vary from simple screening tests which may be easily performed in the office to more complex ones which must be performed in central laboratories or special clinics. Included among the latter are a variety of imaging techniques, as well as microchemical, sialochemical and immunological tests. Some of the tests are non-specific; others, may allow the practitioner to determine the specific cause of the salivary condition. Though the findings in the screening tests are not specific for any disease, they provide ancillary, objective data to support the diagnosis of SGH.

Salivary screening tests

Several, simple salivary screening tests may be performed in the office. Included among these are sialometry, the inspection of the saliva, pH, buffer capacity, and microbiologic assays for lactobacillus and yeast.

Sialometry

Sialometry is the measure of the flow rate of saliva. Whole saliva and/or the secretions from the individual salivary glands, both major and minor, may be collected. Of these, only whole saliva measures overall 'oral wetness'. It is an excellent indicator of the functional status and capacity of the salivary glands and it is simple to collect. The flow rates of both unstimulated and stimulated saliva should be determined. Low UFRs ($\leq$ 0.1 ml/min), indicate that the basal activity of the salivary glands is depressed. A decrease in the flow rate of stimulated saliva indicates that the capacity or ability of the gland to respond to stimuli is decreased. Like other organs, the salivary glands can compensate for a modest loss of parenchyma. Thus, in the early stages of a disease, the SFR may be normal. In later stages, however, low SFRs ($\leq$ 0.5 ml/min) may indicate the presence of damage to the glands. The techniques used to collect whole saliva are described in figure 4.1.

Inspection of saliva

Changes in the physical characteristics of the saliva are commonly observed in patients who suffer from xerostomia. Oftimes, the saliva appears foamy, more viscous and ropy (spinnbarkeit).

Table 4.5 Screening tests: characteristics of whole saliva

Function	Healthy subjects	Patients with severe SGH (eg Sjögren's syndrome or irradiated patients)
Appearance	Serous; slightly foamy; opalescent	Viscous; foamy
Unstimulated flow rate	0.3–0.4 ml/min	Decreased
Stimulated flow rate	1–2 ml/min	Decreased
pH: unstimulated saliva	6.5–6.0	Decreased
Buffer capacity (stimulated saliva)	5.75–6.5	Decreased
Lactobacillus index	< 100 000 cpu/ml (in 55% of population)	Increased
Yeast index	< 100 000 cpu/ml (in 90% of population)	Increased

pH and buffer capacity

Salivary pH and buffer capacity are frequently depressed in patients who complain of oral dryness and suffer from SGH (Table 4.5). The buffer capacity is an indicator of caries susceptibility. These tests can readily be performed in the office by means of pH paper (obtained from chemical supply companies) and buffer capacity indicator strips (Orion Diagnostica, Espoo, Finland).

Microbiological testing

Xerostomia significantly affects the oral flora. The concentration of lactobacilli (indicative of caries susceptibility and sugar intake) and yeast (Candida) often increase (Table 4.5). These changes can be measured in the office with the use of dip slides (Orion Diagnostica, Espoo, Finland). High lactobacillus counts must be viewed with caution, since they are observed in about 45% of the population. But elevated yeast counts are present in only about 10% of normal adults.[20] They are often associated with autoimmune diseases.

Special tests

Collection of saliva from the major and minor salivary glands

Techniques exist to collect and measure the saliva which is secreted from the major and minor salivary glands. The techniques are not difficult,

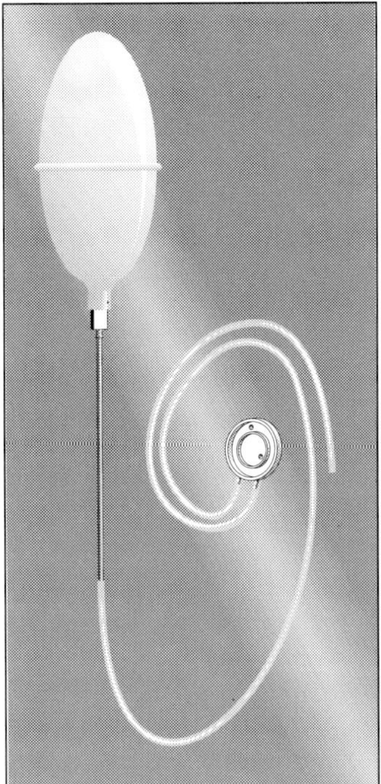

Fig. 4.3 Modified Carlson-Crittenden collector for parotid saliva.

but they require special equipment. A modified Carlson-Crittenden collector is generally employed to collect saliva from the parotid glands (fig. 4.3). It is a two-chambered device. The inner chamber (fig. 4.4) is placed over the orifice of Stenson's duct; thin tubing leads from it to a collecting vessel. The outer chamber is connected by thin tubing to a 'squeeze bulb'. The bulb is compressed and the collector is then placed over the duct opening. Release of the bulb creates suction and causes the device to adhere to the mucosa. Resting or stimulated parotid saliva may be collected. To obtain stimulated parotid saliva, the dorsum of the tongue is swabbed with a 2% citric acid solution.

The combined secretions of the submandibular/sublingual (SM/SL) glands may be easily obtained. Gauze is placed over the orifices of Stenson's ducts to block the secretions from the parotid glands. The secreted, SM/SL saliva, is then aspirated from the floor of the mouth with small, disposable, plastic pipettes.

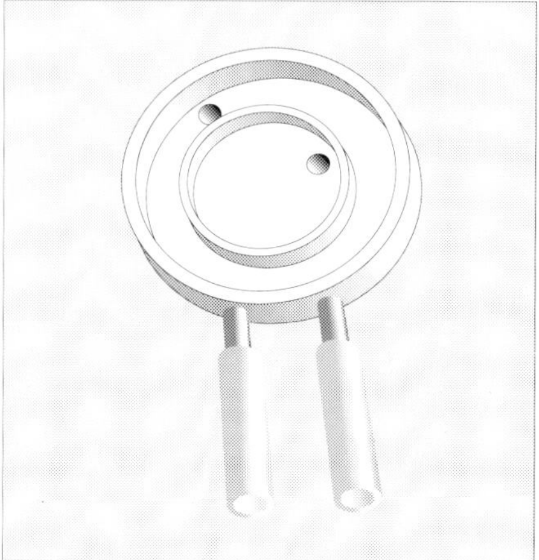

Fig. 4.4 The parotid cup.

Saliva from the minor salivary glands may be measured with the Periotron, an electronic device which measures small (microliter) volumes of fluid by determining its conductivity. The saliva is collected on to small, absorbent paper strips and inserted into the conductivity detector. After calibration the Periotron displays the volume on a digital meter.

Imaging techniques

Sialography is a technique which is primarily used to study the ductal apparatus of the parotid gland. A water or lipid-soluble, iodinated, contrast material is injected into Stenson's duct and its uptake and release are followed by serial roentgenograms, CT or MRI scans. The parotid gland of patients with Sjögren's syndrome frequently exhibit acinar ectasia and extravasation due to acinar atrophy.

Salivary scintigraphy involves the intravenous injection of a radioactive isotope of molybdenum, technetium-99m pertechnetate, and observing its sequential uptake and release from the salivary glands and the thyroid. Decreased uptake and delayed expulsion are associated with salivary gland hypofunction. The technique is particularly useful since it measures the overall function of the parotid and the submandibular glands. However, it is quite expensive and it is questionable whether the findings are superior to those obtained by sialography.

Sialochemistry

Elevated levels of sodium, chloride, and lactoferrin have been observed in the parotid saliva of patients with Sjögren's syndrome[21] and increased concentrations of sodium and IgA have been found in whole saliva.[22] Some of these changes are not specific. The changes in the concentrations of sodium and chloride, for example, may simply be due to a decrease in the volume of water or due to inflammation. On the other hand, the increased concentrations of IgA and lactoferrin have been shown to be due to an actual increase in their synthesis by cells in the salivary glands. The salivary concentrations of many of these substances are quite different from those in blood. Commercial clinical laboratories do not usually adjust their automated machines to measure the salivary levels. As a result, the use of saliva for chemical diagnostic purposes is largely restricted to research laboratories.

Labial or palatal biopsy

The parotid and submandibular glands of patients with Sjögren's syndrome demonstrate acinar atrophy and a characteristic lymphoepithelial infiltrate. Biopsies of the minor salivary glands of the lower lip and the palate reflect the changes observed in the major salivary glands. The diagnosis of Sjögren's syndrome is now largely based on evidence obtained from the labial biopsy.[23]

Immunotesting of whole saliva

The blood of patients with several autoimmune disorders often demonstrate abnormal antibodies. Antinuclear antibodies (ANA) are often observed in systemic lupus erythematosus (SLE), mixed connective tissue disease (MCTD), progressive systemic sclerosis (scleroderma, PSS) and Sjögren's syndrome (SS). Antibodies which are quasi-characteristic of several of these diseases are also observed. Anti Ro (SS-A) and Anti La (SS-B) antibodies are found in SS; Anti Sm and anti RNP antibodies are seen in SLE; and Anti Scl-70 antibodies are present in PSS. Recently, studies have shown that the antibodies associated with Sjögren's syndrome (SS-A/SS-B) and SLE (Anti Sm/RNP) may be detected in the whole saliva of patients with these disorders.[24,25]

The differential diagnosis of xerostomia

As with any diagnosis, a careful history must be taken. Its objective is to determine the nature of the patient's illness and, if possible, its cause. This should enable the dentist or physician to design a rationale course of treatment for the patient.

The provisional diagnosis of SGH can be made if patients complain of oral dryness and there is clinical evidence of disease and abnormal laboratory findings. The medical history can provide information

Table 4.6 Select tests to determine the aetiology of xerostomia and salivary gland hypofunction

Tests for psychological disorders	Tests for lacrimal hypofunction	Blood tests	Imaging tests	Special salivary tests
SCL-90-R	Schirmer's Rose-Bengal	CBC/Diff Rheumatoid factor Antinuclear antibodies (ANA) Anti Ro/SS-A and Anti La/SS-B Anti Sm/RNA Anti Scl-70	X-rays Sialography Salivary scintigraphy CT-Scan MRI	Antibodies (Ab) Anti Ro/SS-A Anti La/SS-A Anti Sm/RNA Anti Scl-70

whether drugs, specific diseases or therapeutic radiation are responsible for the patient's desiccation. The litany of the patient's complaints will indicate whether the changes primarily involve the oral tissues or whether, as is often the case, we are dealing with a serious, generalised exocrinopathy. Further testing is then required to determine the specific cause or causes of the condition. Some of these tests are shown in Table 4.6.

Psychological tests

Patients who profess that their mouth is dry but do not demonstrate clinical or laboratory evidence of disease may be tested for psychological abnormalities with the SCL-90-R Questionnaire. This test is useful in determining the possible role which psychogenic factors may play in the pathogenesis of xerostomia and SGH. The tests consists of 90 questions which the patient must answer. It assays the following functions: depression, anxiety, obsession/compulsion, interpersonal sensitivity, hostility, phobic anxiety, paranoid ideation and psychotropism.

Tests for dry eyes

The Schirmer and Rose-Bengal tests are employed to objectively assess the presence and severity of keratoconjunctivitis sicca (dry eyes) In the Schirmer Test, a standard tear test, filter paper, strips are 'draped' over the lateral portions of the lower lid and left in place for 5 minutes. The strips are then removed and the distance wetted by the secreted ocular fluids is measured. Values less than 5 mm/5 min are considered abnormal. In the Rose-Bengal Test, microliter amounts of the dye are placed in the anterior fornix of each eye. The number of red spots is then estimated in the lateral conjunctiva, the cornea and the nasal conjunctiva. Each region is scored from 0 to 3, and the scores are summed to reveal the Rose-Bengal score for each eye. Scores greater than 3 are considered abnormal.

Blood tests

A mild normocytic, normochromic anemia occurs in many patients with autoimmune diseases; and a large number of them often demonstrate an elevated erythrocyte sedimentation rate (>30 mm/hour, Westergren) and hypergammaglobulinemia. The rheumatoid factor is observed in many patients with rheumatoid arthritis and SS, and antinuclear antibodies are often elevated in many of the rheumatoid diseases. Antinuclear antibody (ANA) levels greater than 1:160 are generally considered abnormal. Abnormal levels of the following antibodies are often associated with the following conditions: 1. Anti Ro/SS-A and/or Anti La/SS-B with Sjögren's syndrome, 2. Anti Sm and Anti RNP with systemic lupus erythematosus and 3. Scl-70 with progressive systemic sclerosis (scleroderma).

The treatment of xerostomia and salivary gland hypofunction

The treatment of xerostomia and SGH is designed to either eliminate the cause or causes of these conditions or, if this is not possible, to alleviate the patients symptoms and clinical signs.

The identification and elimination of the causes of xerostomia and SGH

Since dry mouth is caused by a wide variety of systemic diseases and conditions, it is axiomatic that the identification and cure or amelioration of these disorders will lead to a decrease in the patient's dry mouth feeling, but this is easier said than done. In many instances the desiccation is caused by chronic diseases, like the autoimmune diseases, where, for all practical purposes, there is no cure. In others, it may be due to increasingly severe, irreversible conditions, for example therapeutic irradiation of the head and neck region in the treatment of oral and maxillofacial cancer. On the other hand, the oral dryness which is associated with several forms of dehydration, for example emesis (for example in patients with anorexia nervosa), diarrhoea, or fever are amenable to treatment. So too is the decrease in salivary function due to decreased mastication.

The treatment of drug-induced xerostomia is, likewise, complex. Many commonly used medications possess the capacity to induce oral dryness and SGH (Table 4.3). But the nature and severity of the disease for which these drugs have been prescribed may preclude their removal. It is generally not possible to restrict medications which are employed to treat life-threatening diseases. On the other hand, it may be easy to eliminate the intake of weight-reducing anorectic drugs or the anti-histaminic agents which are often taken to combat the common cold.

The treatment of drug-induced xerostomia involves, in the first instance, the taking of an accurate drug history. Frequently, when presented with the information obtained in the history, the doctor may conclude that one or several of the xerogenic drugs that the patient is taking are no longer necessary or, that the dose of the drug(s) may be lowered. Consideration should also be given to 1. modifying the patient's drug schedule and 2. substituting one xerogenic drug for another, less-drying, one.

The symptomatic treatment of xerostomia and SGH

The objective of these treatments is to increase the overall wetness of the oral tissues. The success of these interventions is dependent on the degree to which the salivary glands are able to respond to various stimuli. In patients with viable, residual salivary gland tissue, it may be possible to stimulate the flow of their saliva. Such patients are referred to as 'responders'. Where this is not possible, in 'non-responders', treatments must be designed to provide moisture to the oral tissues by other means. Sometimes, both methods are employed to relieve oral dryness.

The patient's ability to respond to stimulation may be tested with masticatory or gustatory stimuli. The techniques employed to determine whether the patient is a responder or non-responder are the same as those used to measure the flow of saliva. Paraffin wax is generally employed to test the ability of masticatory stimuli to enhance the flow of saliva; a 2% citric acid solution can be used to determine the effect of chemical stimuli.

The treatment of 'responders'

The following methods are used to promote salivation in responders: 1. masticatory stimuli, 2. chemical stimuli, 3. electronic devices and

4. drugs. In general, patients with xerostomia should be placed on a regimen wherein they alternate various techniques used to simulate flow throughout the day.

Mastication is the normal, physiological, stimulus for salivation. Patients should, therefore, be encouraged to consume foods which require vigorous chewing. Chewing may be made easier if it is accompanied by frequent sips of water. Moreover, they can be advised to increase the number of meals, though not the number of calories, they eat each day. Between meals they should be encouraged to consume low-caloric foods (celery, carrots) or non-foods which require mastication. Keeping a cherry or olive pit in the mouth makes some patients feel better; others use the rind of lemons or oranges. Chewing gum is an extremely effective, rather continuous, sialogogue. Because of the increased risk of dental caries, only the sugarless variety of gum should be used. One study has shown that the frequent chewing of sugarless gum for a period of 2 weeks increased the output of stimulated parotid saliva and increased the pH and buffer capacity of whole and parotid saliva.[26]

Citric acid, present in select fruits and sour and sugarless, 'diabetic' candies or lozenges may also be employed to stimulate the flow of saliva. However, dentate individuals should be advised that acid containing substances, if used frequently or if held in place for long periods of time, as is commonly done, have the capacity to dissolve tooth enamel and make the patient's teeth sensitive to sweets and changes in temperature. Recently, a 2.5% citric acid spray which is saturated with calcium phosphate has been marketed for use in xerostomic patients (ProFlow, ProFlow Corp, Amityville, NY; Optimoist, the Colgate Co.). In vitro tests with ProFlow have demonstrated that this preparation did not demineralise the surfaces of slabs of enamel that were suspended in it for periods up to one week.

An electronic device, which is applied to the tongue and palate, the Salitron (Biosonics Inc., Philadelphia, PA) has been used to stimulate the flow of saliva in patients with Sjögren's syndrome. Those who advocate its use claim that it stimulates flow by augmenting the normal physiologic salivary reflexes.[27] Though an interesting approach to the treatment of dry mouth, there are insufficient data to substantiate its clinical effectiveness.[28]

Several studies have now shown that pilocarpine, 5 mg, tid or qid, is an effective sialogogue in patients with the particularly severe form of xerostomia associated with irradiation for oral and maxillofacial cancer.[29–32] The drug has now been used on some irradiated patients for periods up to three years. Pilocarpine is now being tested on patients with Sjögren's syndrome. This drug provides a useful adjunct to our treatment of xerostomia.

The techniques discussed above depend, for their success, on the presence of functional salivary gland parenchyma. They are, what has been called, intrinsic methods to enhance salivary secretion. An extrinsic approach, which involves salivary replacement therapy, is now being studied at the National Institute of Dental Research in the USA. The vision in this research is to elucidate the mechanisms which control acinar cell proliferation and gene expression. Once known, methods can be devised to increase the number, as well as the activity, of salivary gland cells.[33]

The treatment of non-responders: the use of mouth moisteners

In non-responders, or in those with a minimal response to sialogogues, other methods have to be employed to moisten the oral tissues. The simplest, and perhaps the best of these, is water. Patients, even 'responders', should be told to drink lots of water throughout the day. Moreover, they should be encouraged to carry small bottles of water with them at all times. A plastic bottle, like those used by cyclists, is most helpful. In addition to water, patients should be advised to use room humidifiers, especially at night during the winter months, when rooms tend to be overheated.

A number of substances have been designed to moisten and 'coat' the oral tissues. These are referred to as salivary substitutes or artificial salivas. Saliva, as has been pointed out in Chapter 3, is a complex mixture consisting of water, electrolytes and an elaborate array of organic micro- and macromolecules. Although extensive research is being conducted on the preparation of a 'true' substitute for saliva, none of those currently marketed resemble the 'real thing'.

Commercially available substitutes maybe divided into the following classes: 1. aqueous ion solutions, 2. aqueous-ion and carboxymethylcellulose preparations, 3. mucin-containing solutions, 4. glycoprotein-containing agents and 5. an enzyme-containing gel. Some studies have shown that the aqueous-ion and carboxymethylcellulose preparations were, with the exception of some nocturnal relief, no more effective than a placebo.[34] Clinical trials on Saliva-Orthana, a mucin-containing salivary substitute indicated that patients prefer it to one which contains carboxymethylcellulose. Recent studies suggest that the gel Oral Balance (Laclede Corporation, Gardenia, California, USA) is helpful in dry mouth patients.

Treatment for xerostomia-related oral conditions

Dental caries

Xerostomic patients should be instructed to observe a variety of caries-preventive procedures. Foremost among these is the elimination, or reduction, in the intake of sugars. These should be substituted with substances which are not degraded by oral bacteria into organic acids. Principal among these are sorbitol, xylitol, aspartame, Lycasin and saccharin. The surfaces of the teeth should be treated with fluoride — preparations which contain 0.4% stannous fluoride or 1.1% sodium fluoride can be brushed on to the surfaces of the teeth or applied in a customised tray. Patients should also be taught how to brush their teeth and use dental floss. Carious lesions should be excavated and provisionally restored with temporary restorations. The replacement of these with permanent fillings should be delayed until the caries-activity of the patients is brought under control. Dip slides designed to measure the buffer capacity of saliva (Dentobuff) and the salivary concentrations of *Lactobacillus* (Dentocult) and *Strep. mutans* (Strip Mutans) may be easily employed in the dental office. These are manufactured by Orion Diagnostica (Espoo, Finland).

Dentists should be urged to do everything possible to enhance the patient's ability to masticate foods. This may involve the localised repair of the teeth, periodontal and orthodontic care, the correction of temporomandibular joint dysfunction, the relief of pain, the fabrication of appliances or implants, etc. It should also include dietary counselling.

Candidiasis

Yeast concentrations are frequently elevated in xerostomic patients. Their presence can be diagnosed and monitored by dip-slides designed to culture *Candida albicans* (Oricult-N; Orion Diagnostica, Espoo, Finland). Yeast infections can be treated with a variety of antifungal agents (nystatin, clotrimazole, ketoconazole, fluconazole). Some of these preparations are used locally, as lozenges. Many contain rather high concentrations of sugars and should be used with caution. Fluconzazole is taken *per os*, but it is very expensive. Since the yeast organisms reside on the mucous membranes, it is prudent to advise patients with xerostomia and SGH to regularly brush the dorsum of the tongue and their cheeks. The brushes should be carefully cleaned and stored overnight in a solution of chlorhexidine. So too may the appliances of patients who suffer from denture related candidiasis.

Pain

Pain is not an uncommon finding in patients with oral desiccation, but with the possible exception of the pain associated with obstructed salivary ducts, is not severe. Patients should be taught how to 'milk' the salivary ducts at the first signs of trouble. Some advocate that this should be done regularly, as a prophylactic procedure. Patients with Sjögren's syndrome often state that spicy and/or acidic foods cause oral discomfort; this may be related to the mucosal atrophy alleged to be present in this condition. Once observed, however, they quickly learn to avoid such foods. Sometimes, burning and tingling sensations are particularly troublesome. Such patients may be treated with low doses of select antidepressant medications eg amitriptyline, 25–50 mg/day; diazepam, 2 mg, 2-4 times daily). Localised sore spots, if present, may be treated with a solution of lidocaine HCl (2% to 4%) or dyclonine HCl (0.5% to 1.0%). However, patients should be advised that these analgesic and anesthetic solutions may diminish their ability to distinguish oral sensations, particularly the temperature of hot foods.

Conclusion

Mastication is the normal physiological stimulation for salivation. Besides eating, regular exercise using sugar-free chewing gum can mitigate many of the symptoms related to xerostomia and SGH. But, the fact is, these conditions are due to systemic, often morbid, diseases. Patients who suffer from desiccation are troubled by changes that make their life unpleasant: the pleasures of food, (taste, mastication, swallowing); of phonation and speech; of vision (light sensitivity; blurred vision; burning, itchy and gritty sensations); and even, their self image and sex (dry, cracked lips; dry skin; 'ugly' teeth; dyspareunia) are affected. To put it bluntly, their quality of life is severely diminished. Many equate the generalised desiccation with the fact that life, has come to an end; has 'dried up'! They require expert medical and dental care. But they also need solace, empathy and understanding. In return for such compassion, they offer warmth and appreciation and recognition for a job well done.

References

1 Dawes C. Physiological factors affecting salivary flow rate, oral sugar clearance, and the sensation of dry mouth in man. *J Dent Res* 1987; **66**(Special Issue): 648–653.

2 Shannon I L, Trodahl J N, Starcke E N. Radiosensitivity of the human parotid gland. *Proc Soc Exp Biol Med* 1978; **157:** 50–53.

3 Heft M W, Baum B J. Unstimulated and stimulated salivary flow rate in different age groups. *J Dent Res* 1984; **63:** 1182–1185.
4 Ship J A, Baum B J. Is reduced salivary flow normal in old people? [Letter]. *Lancet* 1990; **336:** 1507.
5 Pedersen W, Schubert M, Izutsu K, Mersai T, Truelove E. Age dependent decreases in human submandibular gland flow rates as measured under resting and post stimulated conditions. *J Dent Res* 1985; **64:** 822–825.
6 Hall H D, Merig J J, Schneyer C A. Metrecal-induced changes in human saliva. *Proc Soc Exp Biol Med* 1967; **124:** 532–536.
7 Sreebny L M, Johnson D A. Effect of food consistency and decreased food intake on the rat parotid and pancreas. *Am J Physiol* 1968; **215:** 455.
8 Menard T, Blomquist D, Izutsu K *et al.* Parotid salivary changes following orthognathic surgery. *J Dent Res* 1985; 64(Spec Issue) Abstract No. 1363, 326.
9 Johnson D A. Regulation of salivary glands and their secretions by masticatory, nutritional and hormonal factors. *In* Sreebny L M (ed) *The salivary system*. Boca Raton: CRC Press, 1987.
10 Sreebny L M, Valdini A. Xerostomia, part I: relationship in other oral syptoms and salivary gland hypofunction. *Oral Surg Oral Med Oral Path* 1988; **66:** 451–458.
11 Kanapka J. Dental diagnostics: a marketing perspective. Speech delivered to the Section on Oral Biology, Amer Assoc Dental Schools, San Francisco, 1989.
12 Billings R J. Studies on the prevalence of xerostomia: Preliminary results. *Caries Res* 1989; **23:** Abstract 124, 35th ORCA Congress.
13 Osterberg T, Landahl S, Hedegard B. Salivary flow, saliva pH and buffering cacity in 70-year-old men and women. *J Oral Rehabil* 1984; **11:** 157–170.
14 Johnson G, Barenthin I, Westpal P. Mouthdryness among patients in long-term hospitals. *Gerodontology* 1984; **3:** 197–203.
15 Thorselius I, Emilson C G, Osterberg T. Salivary conditions and drug consumption in older age groups of elderly Swedish individuals. *Gerodontics* 1988; **4:** 66–70.
16 Narhi T O. Prevalence of subjective feelings of dry mouth in the elderly. *J Dent Res* 1994; **73:** 20–25.
17 Navazesh M, Christensen C M, Brightman V. Clinical criteria for the diagnosis of salivary gland hypofunction. *J Dent Res* 1992; **71:** 1363–1369.
18 Bloch K J, Buchanan W W, Wohl M J. Sjögren's syndrome: a clinical pathological and serological study of 62 cases. *Medicine* 1965; **44:** 187–231.
19 Bertram U. Xerostomia: clinical aspects, pathology and pathogenesis. *Acta Odontol Scand* 1967; **25**(Suppl 49): 126.
20 Parvinen T, Larmas M. The relation of s timulated salivary flow rate and pH to Lactobacillus and yeast concentrations in saliva. *J Dent Res* 1981; **60:** 1929–1935.
21 Stuchel R N, Mandel I D, Baurmash H. Clinical utilisation of sialochemistry in Sjögren's syndrome. *J Oral Pathol* 1984; **13:** 303–309.
22 Ben Aryeh H, Scharf J, Gutman D, Szargel R, Zonis S. Sialochemistry in KCS patients. *Int J Oral Surg* 1978; **7:** 172–177.
23 Daniels T E. Labial salivary gland biopsy in Sjögren's syndrome: Assess-

ment as a diagnostic criterion in 362 suspected cases. *Arth Rheum* 1984; **27:** 147–156.
24 Ben-Chetrit E, Fischel R, Rubinow A. Anti-SSA/RO and anti-SSB/La antibodies in serum and saliva of patients with Sjögren's syndrome. *Clin Rheumatol* 1993; **12:** 471–474.
25 Sreebny L M. The use of whole saliva in the differential diagnosis of Sjögren's syndrome. *Adv Dent Res* 1996; in press.
26 Dodds M W J, Hseih S C, Johnson D A. The effect of increased mastication by daily gum chewing on salivary gland output and dental palque acidogenicity. *J Dent Res* 1991; **70:** 1474–1478.
27 Weiss W W, Brenman H S, Katz P, Bennett J A. Use of an electronic stimulator for the treatment of dry mouth. *J Oral Maxillofac Surg* 1986; **44:** 845–850.
28 US Department of Health and Human Services. AHCPR, Salivary electrostimulation in Sjögren's Syndrome. pp 1–6, March 1991.
29 Fox P C, Van der Ven P F, Baum B J, Mandel I D. Pilocarpine for the treatment of xerostomia associated with salivary gland dysfunction. *Oral Surg Oral Med Oral Path* 1986; **61:** 243–248.
30 Greenspan D, Daniels T E. Effectiveness of pilocarpine in postradiation xerostomia. *Cancer* 1987; **59:** 1123–1125.
31 LeVeque F G, Montgomery M, Potter D *et al.* A multicenter, randomised, double-blind, placebo-controlled, dose-titration study of oral pilocarpine for treatment of radiation-induced xerostomia in head and neck cancer patients. *J Clin Oncol* 1993; **11:** 1124–1131.
32 Johnson J T, Ferretti G A, Nethery W *et al.* Oral pilocarpine for post-irradiation xerostomia in patients with head and neck cancer. *N Engl J Med* 1993; **329:** 390–395.
33 Edgar W M, O'Mullane D M. Treatment of salivary hypofunctions. *In* Edgar W M, O'Mullane D (eds). *Saliva and dental health.* pp 81–88. London: British Dental Journal, 1990.
34 Klestov A C, Webb J, Latt D *et al.* Treatment of xerostomia: a double-blind trial in 108 patients with Sjögren's syndrome. *Oral Surg Oral Med Oral Path* 1981; **51:** 594–599.

5

Clearance of Substances from the Oral Cavity — Implications for Oral Health

Colin Dawes

Differences in the rates of salivary clearance of carbohydrates from food, acids from plaque, and therapeutic substances (for example fluoride) help to explain differences in disease susceptibility among different individuals, and at different sites within a single mouth.

A large number of substances pass through the oral cavity every day, some of which, such as sucrose or acids, are a threat to the health of the mouth, with its unique and vulnerable tissues. Other substances, such as fluoride, may act as a defence, promoting oral health.

Many substances will dissolve in saliva, from which they may then diffuse into, or react with, the oral tissues. The effect of incoming freshly secreted saliva, together with the swallowing process, is to reduce the concentration of dissolved substances, a process that is described as salivary clearance.

Thus, a rapid salivary clearance of harmful substances is beneficial for oral health, while the reverse is true for protective substances.

Models of salivary clearance

The Swenander-Lanke model

The first model of salivary clearance was a simple one suggested by Swenander-Lanke[1] in the mid 1940s. In her model, a chemical (sucrose) dissolves in saliva (of volume V) to create an initial concentration (C_0). Saliva flows at a constant rate (F) into the mouth and is continuously removed (swallowed) at the same rate. The sucrose concentration (C_t) at a later time (t) can be shown to be given by $C_t = C_0.e^{-Ft/V}$. In experimental studies, a graph of the logarithm of the sucrose concentration versus time usually forms a straight line, but only if the plot is begun after the salivary flow rate has returned to the unstimulated rate following the initial rise due to the gustatory stimulation. The rate of

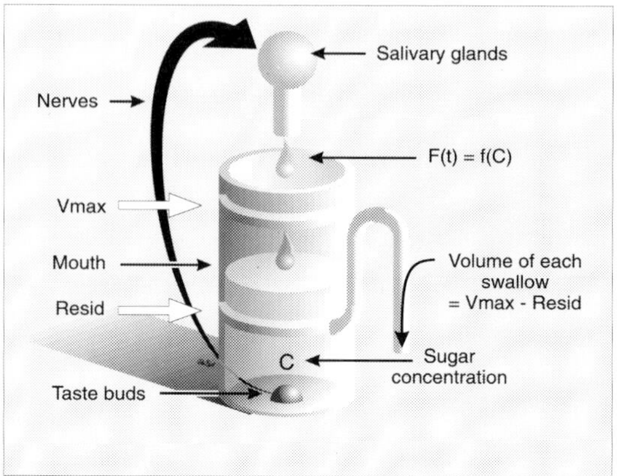

Fig. 5.1 The Dawes (1983) model of oral clearance. Saliva is produced at a rate dependent on the concentration of sugar in the saliva. When a maximum volume of saliva (Vmax) is reached, a swallow occurs and the salivary volume decreases to a residual volume (Resid), thereby eliminating some of the sugar.

decrease in concentration can also be described by using the time taken for the sucrose concentration to decrease by half, or the time taken for the concentration to fall to a given low level.

The Dawes model

A more recent model[2] describes the swallowing process as being equivalent to the action of an incomplete siphon (fig. 5.1). After a swallow, the mouth retains a minimum volume of saliva, called the residual volume. Saliva then flows into the mouth at a rate dependent initially on the stimulating effect of the ingested substance but later, once the concentration is below the taste threshold, or after taste adaptation has occurred, on the unstimulated flow rate. The volume of saliva in the mouth thus increases until a maximum volume is reached. This stimulates the subject to swallow, which clears some of the substance from the oral cavity. The remainder (dissolved in the residual volume of saliva) is then progressively diluted by more saliva entering the mouth until the maximum volume is reached again, and another swallow occurs. The Dawes model has been used to describe with considerable accuracy the clearance of substances, including sucrose, which do not bind to oral surfaces.

Other studies have indicated that with some substances, clearance may occur in two stages, rapidly from the bulk of the saliva, and more slowly from stagnation areas.

Clearance of substances with binding properties

Fluoride

For fluoride, which is a natural component of saliva, and which reacts with the teeth and with plaque, the Dawes model requires further refinement, since plaque fluoride levels can be elevated for several hours following a fluoride rinse or intake of a fluoride tablet and can constitute a 'reservoir' of fluoride.[3]

During the early phase of clearance, when the salivary concentration is still high, some of the fluoride will diffuse into the plaque, or bind to the oral mucosa, from which it is later redistributed back into the bulk saliva. This will delay clearance of fluoride, as will the formation of calcium fluoride deposits on the teeth. These can be formed at higher fluoride concentrations and they will later dissolve slowly. Also, most of the fluoride which is swallowed will be absorbed from the gastrointestinal tract into the blood and then a very small fraction of this (< 0.2%) will be recycled via the salivary glands. When all of these factors are built into a computer model, it is possible to evaluate the effects of a single variable on clearance while keeping other variables constant.[4]

Chlorhexidine

Chlorhexidine, in the form of rinses, gels, or varnishes, is an antibacterial agent used for plaque control and for the prevention of both dental caries and periodontitis. An important property (termed substantivity) of chlorhexidine is its ability to bind more strongly than other antibacterial substances to the oral surfaces. This greatly delays its clearance from the mouth, thereby prolonging its effectiveness.

Micro-organisms

Not only may micro-organisms bind to oral surfaces but they may also proliferate there. Since whole saliva may contain as many as 10^9 bacteria/ml, salivary clearance plays an important role in removing bacteria from the mouth and individuals with xerostomia will have higher salivary bacterial counts (see Chapter 4).

After a prophylaxis, and in the subsequent absence of oral hygiene, the amount of plaque on the teeth and micro-organisms on the oral mucosa will gradually increase until an equilibrium is reached when the rate at which bacteria are being shed into saliva is equal to the rate of their proliferation on the oral surfaces. At that time, the lower the

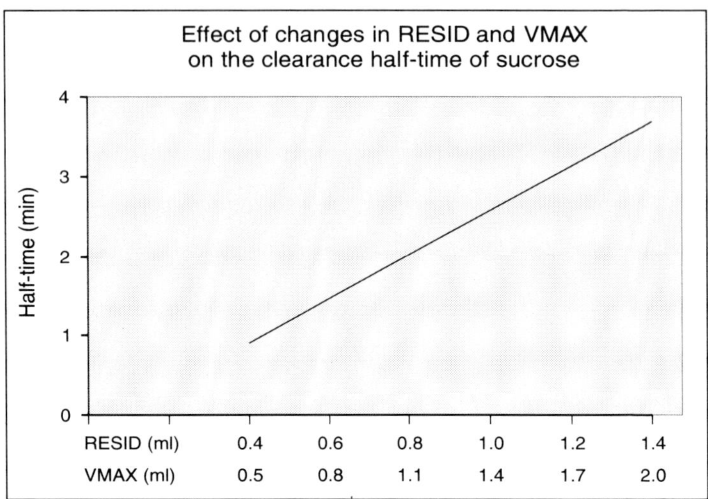

Fig. 5.2 A computer simulation of the effect of changes in the residual volume after swallowing (Resid) and the maximum volume before swallowing (Vmax) on the clearance halftime of sucrose after a 10% sucrose mouthrinse. The clearance halftime is the time for the concentration to fall by half.

salivary flow rate, the higher will be the salivary bacterial count. Since salivary flow is very low during sleep (see Chapter 3), this explains why the salivary bacterial count, and incidentally the tendency to halitosis, is greatest before breakfast.

Some factors influencing salivary clearance

The most important variables are the residual and maximum volumes, the unstimulated and stimulated flow rates, and the extent to which the substance being cleared binds to oral surfaces.[5]

The volume of saliva left in the mouth after swallowing (residual volume)

As measured in studies on 40 normal individuals,[6] the mean residual volume is about 0.8 ml, but the large range (0.4–1.4 ml) suggests that variations in the residual volume may be responsible for some individual differences in clearance patterns. According to the Dawes computer model, the effect of varying the residual volume on clearance half-time (the time for the salivary sucrose concentration to decrease by half) after a 10% sucrose mouthrinse is very large (fig. 5.2). In fact, the difference in concentration obtained with the lowest residual volume (0.4 ml) and the highest volume tested (1.4 ml) was more than 50-fold after only ten minutes. Thus individuals who swallow more effectively (ie have a low residual volume) will clear substances from the mouth more quickly.

The volume of saliva in the mouth just prior to swallowing (maximum volume)

Another important physiological variable affecting salivary clearance is the maximum volume of saliva allowed to accumulate in the mouth before swallowing is initiated. The mean value in 40 individuals was 1.1 ml, but as with the residual volume, a wide range (0.5–2.1 ml) was found, those with larger residual volumes naturally having larger maximum volumes.[6] Again, a large effect on the clearance half-time is seen (fig. 5.2), and individuals who do not allow as much saliva to accumulate in the mouth before swallowing will clear the substance more rapidly.

The unstimulated salivary flow rate

The unstimulated salivary flow rate is normally about 0.3 ml/minute but may vary a great deal among individuals (see Chapter 3). Since the swallowing frequency is dependent on the rate of entry of saliva into the mouth, it is obvious that the salivary flow rate is an extremely important variable. According to the Dawes model, the lower the unstimulated salivary flow rate, the more prolonged will be the clearance half-time for sucrose (fig. 5.3). Since individuals with severe xerostomia may have unstimulated flow rates even lower than the minimum value of 0.05 ml/minute shown in the figure, the delayed clearance of carbohydrate may help to account for their high susceptibility to dental caries.

The stimulated salivary flow rate

Although salivary flow may remain above the unstimulated rate for only about a minute after food consumption or after a sucrose rinse, the initial rate at which the sucrose is diluted plays a critical role in determining how much sucrose diffuses into dental plaque. The longer the salivary sucrose concentration remains high, the more sucrose will diffuse into dental plaque. In individuals with a normal unstimulated flow rate, the salivary sucrose concentration will have fallen so low within the first two or three minutes after a sucrose rinse that a rinse with water at that time would have little influence on acid production in plaque.

Lagerlöf has also shown, in a computer model, that the stimulated flow rate can have a great effect on the clearance pattern of fluoride.[4] As with sucrose, the faster clearance rate caused by stimulation of salivary flow reduces the amount of fluoride diffusing into dental plaque.

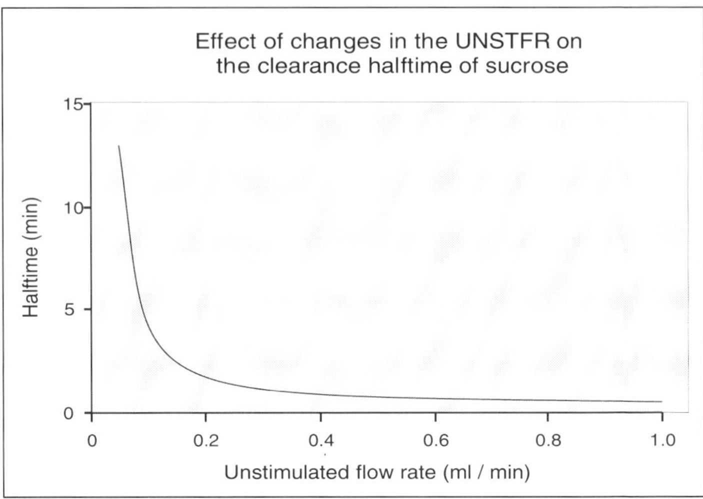

Fig. 5.3 A computer simulation of the effect of changes in the unstimulated flow rate on the clearance of sucrose after a 10% sucrose mouthrinse. The simulation assumed average values for Resid (0.8 ml), and Vmax (1.1 ml).

In formulating cariostatic topical fluoride products, such as fluoride tablets, it thus seems advisable to use agents which do not stimulate salivation, in other words, ones that are tasteless, and allow them to dissolve slowly in the mouth rather than be chewed.

Saliva as a film

For too long, oral biologists have generally thought of dental plaque as being covered by a large volume of saliva, the composition of which remains essentially constant unless the flow rate changes. In fact, for most of the time, saliva is present as a very thin film whose composition changes locally when materials diffuse into or out of dental plaque. Given an average volume of saliva in the mouth of about 1 ml, and that the surface area of the adult mouth is just over 200 cm^2, the saliva must be present as a film averaging about 0.1 mm or less in thickness.[7] When flow is unstimulated the film has been estimated to move at different rates (0.8-8 mm/minute) in different regions of the mouth.[8] These extremely slow velocities have important implications for the clearance of ingested carbohydrate and topical fluoride, but particularly for clearance of acid from dental plaque. Figure 5.4 shows the postulated directions of flow of the salivary film.

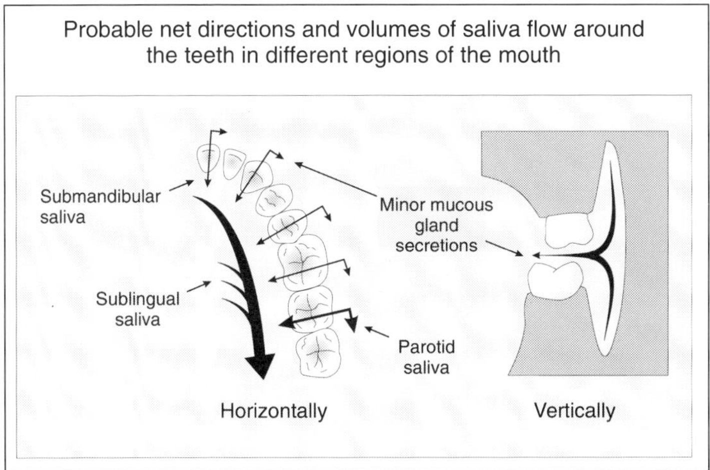

Fig. 5.4 Diagrammatic representation of the anticipated directions and volumes of salivary flow in different locations in the mouth.

Clearance of substances from local sites

Ingested carbohydrate

Dental caries is caused by the demineralising effects of organic acids produced in dental plaque by micro-organisms that ferment carbohydrates, most notably sucrose. The Stephan curve is the fall and subsequent rise in plaque pH which occurs after exposure of dental plaque to fermentable carbohydrate. In regions of the mouth where clearance is rapid, less sucrose will be available to diffuse into dental plaque, and thus less acid will be formed.

Studies by Lagerlöf and co-workers,[9,10] Weatherell and colleagues,[11] and Dawes and Macpherson[12,13] have shown that sucrose ingested in several different forms is distributed very unevenly around the mouth and is cleared at very different rates in different locations. In general, clearance is more rapid from lingual than from buccal tooth surfaces, except buccal to the upper molars where parotid saliva enters the mouth. Apart from that region, buccal tooth surfaces are mostly exposed to the extremely viscous secretions from the minor mucous glands. In contrast, lingual surfaces are exposed mainly to the secretions from two of the major salivary glands, namely the submandibular and sublingual.

Figure 5.5 illustrates mean results on 10 subjects for the clearance of sucrose from whole saliva and from six specific oral sites after a 10%

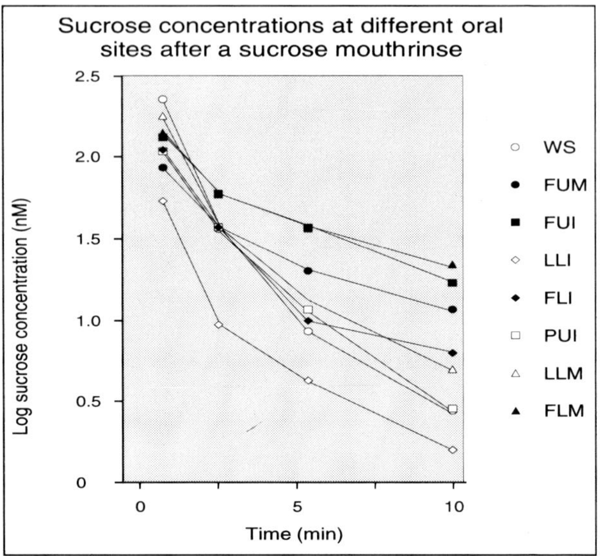

Fig. 5.5 Sucrose concentrations in saliva at different sites and times after a 10% sucrose mouthrinse. WS = whole saliva; FUM = facial upper molars; FUI = facial upper incisors; LLI = lingual lower incisors; FLI = facial lower incisors; PUI = palatal upper incisors; LLM = lingual lower molars; FLM = facial lower molars.

sucrose mouthrinse.[12] Because the ordinate is a logarithmic scale, a change of one unit represents a ten-fold change in concentration. The higher the salivary film velocity in a given region, the lower is the initial concentration of sucrose and the more rapid is its clearance. Compare, for instance, clearance from the lingual of the lower incisors with that from the facial of the lower molars, where the salivary film velocities, when flow is unstimulated, have been estimated to average 8 mm/minute and 1 mm/minute, respectively.

Topical fluoride

The current view of fluoride's role in demineralisation and remineralisation of enamel stresses the value of raising the fluoride level in the liquid surrounding the enamel crystals slightly and for prolonged periods of time. To be effective, only a small increase in salivary fluoride concentration is needed above the normal value of about 1 µmol/l (0.019 ppm). This certainly occurs during, and for a certain time after, the use of dentifrices, which usually contain about 1000 ppm F, and during other preventive applications of fluoride. Those sites where the salivary film velocity is low have been shown by Weatherell and his colleagues[14]

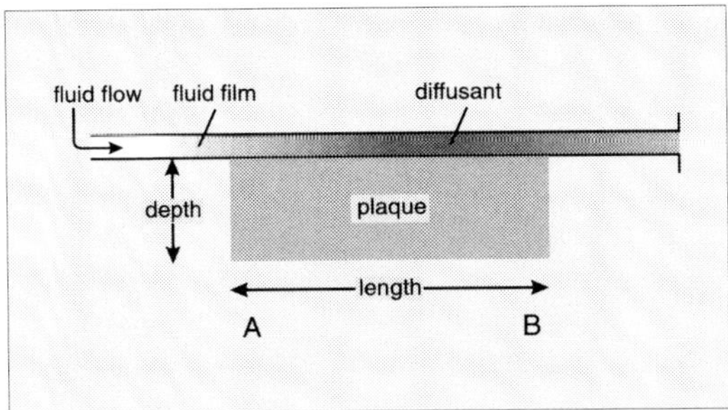

Fig. 5.6 Diagrammatic representation of the flow of a slowly-moving film of saliva over dental plaque and the accumulation of a diffusant (such as organic acid) in the film at the distal edge of the plaque.

to clear fluoride more slowly, which will facilitate its anticariogenic action at the sites most susceptible to caries.

Acid from dental plaque

When plaque is exposed to sugar, the bacteria in plaque form acid which will tend to diffuse toward the tooth surface but also out of the plaque, down its concentration gradient into saliva. A computer model of this process[15] suggested that if the salivary film is moving slowly over plaque, acid will accumulate in the film and reduce the concentration gradient between the plaque and the saliva, which will retard the diffusion of acid out of the plaque (fig. 5.6). These predictions of the computer model were tested in a physical model[16] in which 10% sucrose was passed for 1 minute over a 0.5-mm deep artificial plaque of *Streptococcus oralis* (with the same acid-forming ability and buffering capacity as natural plaque), followed by unstimulated saliva at three different film velocities and with a film thickness of 0.1 mm. The film velocities of 0.8 and 8 mm/min are, respectively, the lowest and highest mean values estimated in the mouth when salivary flow is unstimulated, while 86 mm/min is about ten times higher than the latter. The resulting Stephan curves (fig. 5.7) at positions A and B (see Fig. 5.6) on the undersurfaces of the plaque were much deeper and more prolonged at the lowest film velocity, especially at position B. Thus oral regions with a more slowly moving salivary film (eg buccal to the upper incisors — velocity 0.8 mm/minute) might be more susceptible to caries than regions with a faster moving salivary film (eg lingual to the lower incisors — velocity 8 mm/minute) because acid is cleared away from plaque more slowly at a low film velocity.

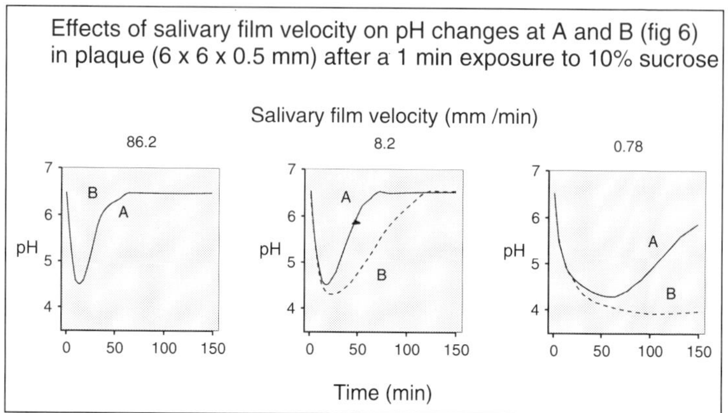

Fig. 5.7 Effect of fluid film velocity on the pH at position A (see fig. 5.6), where the plaque is first contacted by fresh saliva, and at position B (see fig. 5.6), where the salivary film leaves the plaque, under an artificial plaque 6 mm square and 0.5 mm deep after exposure to a 10% sucrose solution for 1 minute.

The effect on the Stephan curve of a mouthrinse with water

It has often been reported that rinsing the mouth with water after eating or drinking sugary items does not significantly reduce the fall in plaque pH, suggesting perhaps that the role of saliva in the clearance of sugar and in the clearance of plaque acid, by diffusion into saliva, has been overestimated. By contrast, stimulation of salivary flow by the chewing of sugar-free chewing gum, which increases the bicarbonate concentration in saliva, is very effective in restoring plaque pH to neutrality. This could suggest that the salivary effect is due only to the buffering power of the bicarbonate in saliva, rather than to the enhanced clearance of sugar or acid.

However, the lack of effect of mouthrinsing with water on the Stephan curve may be partly because it is generally done too late: two minutes after a sucrose challenge, the sugar concentration in saliva is usually lower than that in plaque, so rinsing with water at that time would not be expected to reduce the diffusion of sugar into plaque, unless the sugar clearance were excessively slow, as in xerostomic subjects. As far as the removal of acid is concerned, outward diffusion of hydrogen ions alone does not adequately explain plaque neutralisation. Shellis and Dibdin[17] have shown that most of the H^+ ions in dental plaque are fixed to bacterial surface proteins and other fixed buffers. That is why mobile salivary buffers such as bicarbonate and phosphate, which are present in the salivary film (but not in a water rinse), are so important. They are able to diffuse into plaque as HCO_3^- and HPO_4^{2-}

ions, capture the hydrogen ions from the fixed buffers, and diffuse out into the saliva as H_2CO_3 and as $H_2PO_4^-$ ions.

The advantage of mouthrinsing after meals is that it also helps to remove food debris as well as sugars in solution and this may be particularly valuable in individuals with xerostomia in whom sugar clearance may be greatly delayed (see fig. 5.3).

The site-specificity of dental caries and calculus deposition

In a fasted subject, the extracellular fluid phase of dental plaque (plaque fluid) is normally supersaturated with respect to several calcium phosphates, such as those in teeth and dental calculus. This condition favours remineralisation of early caries lesions and deposition of calculus. However, when plaque is exposed to fermentable carbohydrate, the bacteria form acid, and if the pH falls below a critical value (probably about 5.1–5.5), the plaque fluid becomes unsaturated. At such times, the teeth will tend to dissolve (dental caries), as will the calcium phosphate crystals present in early calculus.

Dawes and Macpherson[12] have postulated that supragingival calculus forms most readily on the lingual surfaces of the lower anterior teeth and the buccal surfaces of the upper molars because these are sites with a high salivary film velocity. This will promote the development of shallow Stephan curves, because of the rapid clearance of sugar from the adjacent saliva and because of the rapid clearance of acid from dental plaque, and there will be little opportunity for calcium phosphate crystals in early calculus to dissolve during meals or snacks. They have also suggested that smooth-surface caries is much more prevalent buccally than lingually because salivary film velocity is much lower buccally than lingually. A low film velocity buccally will slow the rate of sucrose clearance from the saliva and the clearance of acid from dental plaque, which will promote the development of deep and prolonged Stephan curves and enamel dissolution, leading to dental caries.

The mouth is clearly not a uniform environment but contains many distinct microenvironments, some of which are more conducive than others to the development of oral disease.

Summary — Clinical Highlights

Rapid oral clearance of micro-organisms, of sucrose and other carbohydrate substrates, and of acid from plaque metabolism, will be of clinical benefit. However, for protective agents like fluoride or chlorhexidine, a slow clearance is preferable. Knowledge of the factors determining clearance rates in different locations is leading to a more detailed picture of the reasons for the site-specificity of dental caries and supragingival calculus deposition and of how to maximise some benefits - for example, the avoidance of salivary stimulation with topical fluoride applications and by allowing fluoride tablets to dissolve slowly in the mouth rather than be chewed.

Acknowledgement

Thanks are due to Dr. F. Lagerlöf, who gave the original presentation which formed the basis for Chapter 7 in the First Edition. We thank the *Journal of Dental Research* for permission to include Fig. 5.4 (Fig. 3 from *J Dent Res* **66:** 1614–1618, 1987).

Further reading

1 Swenander-Lanke L. Influence on salivary sugar of certain properties of foodstuffs and individual oral conditions. *Acta Odontol Scand* 1957; **15:** Supplement 23.
2 Dawes C. A mathematical model of salivary clearance of sugar from the oral cavity. *Caries Res* 1983; **17:** 321–334.
3 Aasenden R, Brudevold F, Richardson B. Clearance of fluoride from the mouth after topical treatment or the use of a fluoride mouthrinse. *Arch Oral Biol* 1968; **13:** 625–636.
4 Lagerlöf F, Oliveby A, Ekstrand J. Physiological factors influencing salivary clearance of sugar and fluoride. *J Dent Res* 1987; **66:** 430–435.
5 Dawes C. Physiological factors affecting salivary flow rate, oral sugar clearance, and the sensation of dry mouth in man. *J Dent Res* 1987; **66:** 648–653.
6 Lagerlöf F, Dawes C. The volume of saliva in the mouth before and after swallowing. *J Dent Res* 1984; **63:** 618–621.
7 Collins L M C, Dawes C. The surface area of the adult human mouth and thickness of the salivary film covering the teeth and oral mucosa. *J Dent Res* 1987; **66:** 1300–1302.
8 Dawes C, Watanabe S, Biglow-Lecomte P, Dibdin G H. Estimation of the velocity of the salivary film at some different locations in the mouth. *J Dent Res* 1989; **68:** 1479–1482.
9 Britse A, Lagerlöf F. The diluting effect of saliva on the sucrose concentration in different parts of the human mouth after a mouth-rinse with sucrose. *Arch Oral Biol* 1987; **32:** 755–756.
10 Lindfors B, Lagerlöf F. Effect of sucrose concentration in saliva after a sucrose rinse on the hydronium ion concentration in dental plaque. *Caries Res* 1988; **22:** 7–10.
11 Weatherell J A, Duggal M S, Robinson C, Curzon M E J. Site-specific differences in human dental plaque pH after sucrose rinsing. *Arch Oral Biol* 1988; **33:** 871–873.
12 Dawes C, Macpherson L M. The distribution of saliva and sucrose around the mouth during the use of chewing gum and the implications for the site-specificity of caries and calculus deposition. *J Dent Res* 1993; **72:** 852–857.

13 Macpherson L M D, Dawes C. Distribution of sucrose around the mouth and its clearance after a sucrose mouthrinse or consumption of three different foods. *Caries Res* 1994; **28:** 150–155.
14 Weatherell J A, Strong M, Robinson C, Ralph J P. Fluoride distribution in the mouth after fluoride rinsing. *Caries Res* 1986; **20 :** 111–119.
15 Dawes C. An analysis of factors influencing diffusion from dental plaque into a moving film of saliva and the implications for caries. *J Dent Res* 1989; **68:** 1483–1488.
16 Macpherson L M D, Dawes C. Effects of salivary film velocity on pH changes in an artificial plaque containing *Streptococcus oralis*, after exposure to sucrose. *J Dent Res* 1991; **70:** 1230–1234.
17 Shellis R P, Dibdin G H. Analysis of the buffering systems in dental plaque. *J Dent Res* 1988; **67:** 438–446.

6
Saliva and the Control of Plaque pH

Michael Edgar and Susan M Higham

The Stephan curve

Acidogenic bacteria in dental plaque can rapidly metabolise certain carbohydrates to acid end-products. In the mouth, the resultant change in plaque pH over time is called a Stephan curve (fig. 6.1). Under resting conditions the pH is fairly constant although intersubject differences between individuals, and between sites in one individual are found. Following exposure of the plaque to fermentable carbohydrate the pH decreases rapidly to reach a minimum after approximately 5–20 minutes before slowly returning to its starting value over 30–60 minutes.

Resting plaque pH

The term 'resting plaque' refers to plaque 2–2.5 hours after the last intake of dietary carbohydrate as opposed to 'starved plaque' which has not been exposed to carbohydrates for 8–12 hours. Resting plaque pH is usually between 6 and 7 whereas the starved plaque pH is normally between 7 and 8. A large range of plaque pH values seem to be compatible with oral health, but due to the multifactorial nature of dental caries, what may be healthy for one individual may be unhealthy for another.

Resting plaque contains relatively high concentrations of acetate compared with lactate. The predominant amino acids are glutamate and proline, with ammonia also found at significant levels.[1] The presence of elevated levels of acetate is due to the accumulation of end products of amino acid breakdown as well as those of carbohydrate metabolism. These metabolic products are present at much higher concentrations than in saliva. This is partly due to the fact that they are constantly produced from the metabolism of intracellular and extracellular bacterial carbohydrate stores, and from the breakdown of salivary

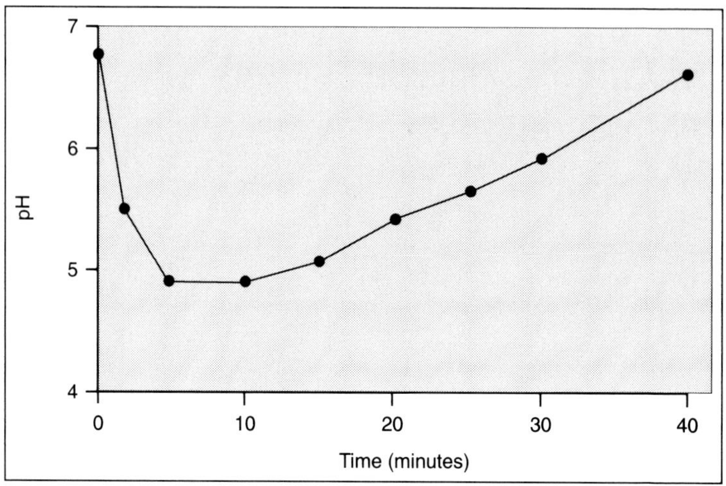

Fig. 6.1 Diagram of a Stephan curve — the plaque pH response to a 10% glucose solution (Redrawn from Jenkins, *The physiology and biochemistry of the mouth*. Blackwell, London, 1978).

glycoproteins. Their diffusion out of plaque is hindered by the slow salivary film velocity (Chapter 5) under 'resting' conditions when saliva is unstimulated.

The decrease in plaque pH

Two main factors affect the rate at which the pH decreases:

1. the presence of exogenous, rapidly fermentable carbohydrate, usually sugars.

2. low buffering capacity of saliva at unstimulated salivary flow rates.

The fall in pH has been principally related to the production of lactate.[2] Simultaneously acetate and propionate are lost from the plaque. These acids were thought to be lost to saliva but more recent work has indicated that they may also diffuse from the plaque into the tooth.[3] In terms of pH change in plaque, the amount of a low pK acid such as lactate relative to a higher pK acid such as acetate is very important. The high pK acids provide a buffering system because they can absorb the hydrogen ions generated by dissociation of the low pK acids.[4] It is possible that the fall in pH is enhanced by a reduction of plaque buffering power due to acetate. The nature of the acids in plaque may be important because they differ in their ability to attack enamel. As the pH of plaque decreases the concentration of amino acids and ammonia in plaque also fall rapidly.[1] This fall may be due to the uptake and utilisation of nitrogenous material for anabolic reactions stimulated by the availability of energy from carbohydrate fermentation.

The minimum plaque pH

The minimum value of plaque pH and how long the pH stays at that minimum is determined by several factors:

1. whether any fermentable carbohydrate remains in the mouth, and whether the carbohydrate has been cleared for example, by swallowing, rather than being metabolised by bacteria.

2. the pH may fall to values at which bacterial enzyme systems cease to function properly.

3. the buffering capacity, both in plaque and saliva, but particularly in stimulated saliva, may be critical.

The minimum pH corresponds with the greatest concentration of lactate produced during a Stephan curve and with a reduction in acetate, succinate, propionate, most of the amino acids and ammonia. The length of time that the pH remains at its minimum is important since if it reaches the so called 'critical pH' which is the pH at which saliva and plaque fluid cease to be saturated with respect to calcium and phosphate, then conditions may be reached which permit the dissolution of the enamel (Chapter 9).

The rise in plaque pH

The steady rise in pH back to the resting value is influenced by all the factors mentioned above, including diffusion of acids out of the plaque into saliva. It is also influenced by base production in plaque. Ammonia is highly alkaline, neutralises acid and causes a rise in pH. It is a predominant basic constituent of plaque fluid and is also present in saliva. It is derived mainly from the breakdown of urea but also from the deamination of amino acids particularly arginine and arginine peptides.[5] Decarboxylation reactions in plaque result in the formation of amines leading to pH rise. These reactions are thought to have a significant neutralising effect in plaque under conditions of moderate carbohydrate intake but not when intake is frequent. Glutamate has been found to be the predominant amino acid in the majority of plaque fluid samples taken during a Stephan curve.[1] A number of bacteria are able to synthesise glutamate from carbohydrate. Glutamate is an extremely important amino acid since it is able to act as an amino donor in the synthesis of most amino acids, all of which are less acidic than the organic acids. Delta-amino-n-valeric acid (DAVA), a basic component, has been detected in plaque from monkeys[6] and in humans where its minimum concentration coincided with the pH minimum following sucrose rinsing.[1] DAVA production is associated with proline reduction via the Stickland reaction (Chapter 7). DAVA is potentially an important pH regulator in plaque, not only because its formation may divert reduced nicotinamide adenine dinucleotide (NAD) from lactate synthesis, but also because of the basicity associated with its free amino group. Acid neutralising mechanisms in plaque may also be derived from the removal of acids by the conversion of lactate to weaker organic acids. Bacteria belonging to the genus Veillonella metabolise lactate to less acidic products. Some of the acetate and lactate will also be lost by diffusion into enamel. The breakdown of carbohydrates stored by bacteria within plaque may also slow the pH rise.

Thirty minutes following the consumption of fermentable carbohydrate, the pH is almost back to its resting level. However the organic acid profile (the proportion of different organic acids such as lactate and acetate in plaque) does not return to resting levels until much later.

Maintenance of plaque pH by saliva

Many years ago, researchers compared the Stephan curves produced following a sucrose rinse, with and without salivary restriction. The results showed that excluding saliva by cannulating the ducts of the major glands and diverting the saliva outside the mouth, lowered the minimum pH and slowed recovery to the baseline pH (fig. 6.2).

Saliva is very important in maintaining a neutral pH in plaque and in the oral cavity. Its ability to perform this function can largely be attributed to bicarbonate and to a lesser extent to phosphate as well as other factors.

Bicarbonate

This is the most important buffering system in stimulated saliva. Metabolically derived bicarbonate increases with salivary gland activity, so that bicarbonate provides an increasingly effective buffer system against acid, especially at high flow rates when concentrations may reach up to 60 mM. Salivary pH also rises with the increase in flow rate, so in addition to its buffering effect, stimulated saliva neutralises plaque acidity.

Phosphate

The phosphate system has an important role at low salivary flow rates. In unstimulated saliva concentrations may peak at around 10 mM. This system is however of minor importance in stimulated saliva because of the fall in phosphate concentration at high rates of flow. Phosphate has

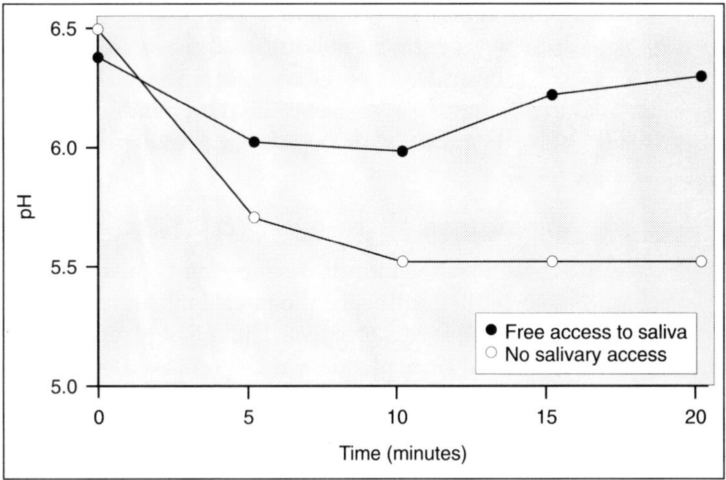

Fig. 6.2 The effect of restricting the access of saliva to plaque upon the shape of the Stephan curve (Reproduced from Jenkins, *The physiology and biochemistry of the mouth*. Blackwell, London, 1978)

a protective role due in part to its ability to maintain the saturation of saliva with these ions which favours the integrity of the mineral phase of the teeth.

Other factors

Saliva contains urea at concentrations similar to those in blood. Many plaque organisms posses urease activity, converting urea to ammonia, thus raising plaque pH. Saliva also contains other substances which have the ability to increase pH known as pH rise factors. The most well known of these is sialin, and has been identified as a basic peptide containing arginine.[7] These factors exert their effect by stimulating base production by oral bacteria. Some bacteria can decarboxylate the amino acids from salivary peptides to form amines; these are alkaline and also remove hydrogen ions from the system. Base production is responsible for the fact that the pH of starved plaque is often higher than that of the saliva bathing it.

Buffering capacity of plaque

Plaque has an intrinsic 'fixed' buffering capacity, due mainly to bacterial proteins and other macromolecules in plaque. These fixed buffers are in equilibrium with 'mobile' buffers — phosphates and bicarbonate — which exchange with those in saliva (Chapter 5).

Calcium phosphate crystals are thought to be present even in young plaque and can dissolve under acid conditions to increase greatly the buffering capacity. This can also raise the concentrations of calcium and phosphate ions, and thus help to oppose the demineralisation of the tooth. A negative correlation exists between calcium phosphates in plaque, and caries activity.[8]

Age and site of plaque

The age and site of plaque in the mouth are important considerations in plaque pH studies since they influence the microbial composition and thickness of plaque and the access of saliva. The age of plaque is usually defined as the time elapsed since plaque was last removed, for example, by scaling or very thorough home toothcleaning. But this definition is limited because plaque is always being disturbed and removed by the action of the tongue and cheeks and by foods. The thickness of plaque, therefore, is probably more important. Thickness affects microbial composition and how easily substances can diffuse through plaque. Thicker plaques are more anaerobic, and so in the inner layers will favour the growth of strictly anaerobic species. The rate of penetration of nutrients will depend on the cube of the thickness of the plaque, and also on whether the nutrient molecule has negative or positive charged groups. Calcium and phosphate levels in plaque increase with time; 10-day-old plaque has about 25% of the mineral content of calculus. Most plaque pH studies use plaque from subjects who have refrained from oral hygiene procedures for 24 or 48 hours.

It is sometimes suggested that toothbrushing may be more effective before meals, because the residual plaque is too thin to lead to a large pH drop, and if fluoride dentifrice is used, plaque metabolism will be inhibited. However, the salivary stimulation during eating is known to accelerate the clearance of fluoride from the mouth, and this disadvantage may outweigh the possible advantages of brushing before meals.

Diet history

The dietary history of plaque is one of the most important factors affecting the Stephan curve. Even a modest restriction of sugar intake for 1–2 days will considerably influence the shape of the curve. For example, when plaque pH in humans is compared before and after a sequence of sucrose rinses over 3 weeks, there will be a decrease in both the resting pH and the minimum pH. Many oral micro-organisms produce extracellular polysaccharides in the presence of excess sucrose. These include extracellular glucans which are thought to increase plaque adhesion and thickness, as well as extracellular fructans which are subsequently broken down to acid. Some micro-organisms build up intracellular polysaccharide stores, the breakdown of which is an ongoing contribution to acid production in resting plaque.

Plaque pH and salivary clearance

Salivary clearance rate is a term used to describe the dilution and removal of substrates and acids from the mouth (see chapter 5). The flow rate of saliva has the greatest influence on the rate of clearance — the higher the flow, the faster the clearance rate. Patients with rapid clearance rates have a shallow Stephan curve whereas those who clear more slowly have deeper curves since lower pH values are reached.[9] Studies have shown that the labial and upper anterior region is a site of slow clearance, the lingual and lower anterior region is a site of rapid clearance, and the buccal area a site of intermediate clearance. The plaque pH in these regions relates well to the rate of clearance. The approximal surfaces of the upper anteriors have the lowest plaque pH, since clearance is slower from these sites. This also relates to the caries prevalence in anterior teeth, being higher in upper than lower approximal surfaces (Chapter 5). A significant positive correlation between the residual volume of saliva and the caries experience of an individual has been found.[10] The residual volume is important in determining the clearance rate: the smaller the volume, the faster the clearance.

Plaque pH in renal dialysis patients

Children on renal dialysis have high concentrations of ammonia and urea in saliva compared with normal children. In one study it was found that although the children on dialysis ate many sweets, they had a lower caries experience than the control children. It is likely that this is due to a direct effect of salivary urea and ammonia on plaque pH, as plaque from these children was capable of forming acid from sugars.[11]

Plaque pH and fluoride levels

Salivary fluoride levels, even in a fluoridated area and after using fluoride toothpaste, are quite low, about 0.5–2.0 µmol/l (0.01–0.04 parts/10^6). It has been shown that an increased systemic intake of fluoride will lead to an elevated level of plasma fluoride and subsequently raised salivary levels. This can lead to increases in plaque fluoride level. It is also known that a high level of fluoride is retained in plaque for up to 8 hours after a fluoride rinse. Fluoride levels in plaque are usually 50–100 times higher than that in whole saliva.

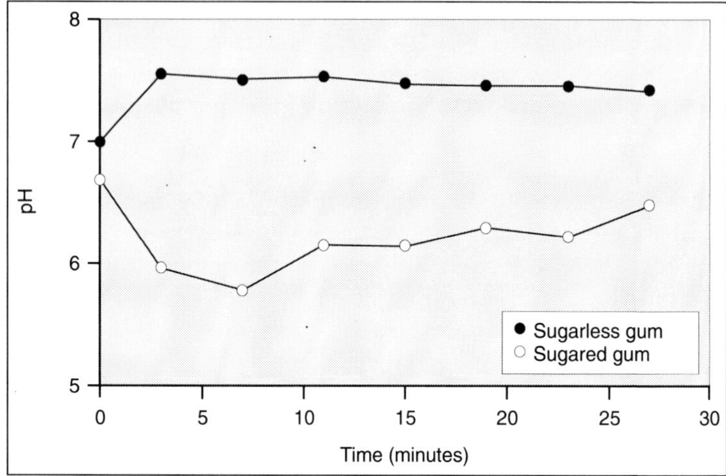

Fig. 6.3 Plaque pH responses to chewing sugarless or sugared chewing gum (Reproduced from Rugg-Gunn *et al.*, *Br Dent J* 1978; **145:** 95-100).

Systemic fluorides have only a small effect on plaque acid production, but their effect may be great enough to tip the scales between demineralisation and remineralisation of tooth enamel. Part of the fluoride in plaque is present in a bound form, but part is released into solution when the pH falls. This can also be potentially beneficial in favouring remineralisation and modifying subsequent bacterial metabolism. Topically administered fluorides have antibacterial actions but this is a direct effect and not mediated by saliva. However, fluoride from dentifrices, gels and other vehicles may bind to the soft tissues or precipitate on the tooth surface as calcium fluoride, which then slowly dissolves into the saliva and elevates the salivary fluoride concentration slightly.

Salivary stimulation and plaque pH

The knowledge that saliva is beneficial in terms of plaque pH and buffering following consumption of a cariogenic food, has produced much interest in agents which stimulate an increase in salivary flow. Chewing gum has been tested in plaque pH studies with sugar-free gum producing a rise in plaque pH reflecting the raised pH of stimulated saliva. With a sugar-containing gum, despite a stimulated salivary flow, there was a decrease in pH which lasted for 20 minutes (fig. 6.3). Chewing would therefore seem to have a beneficial effect on plaque pH by promoting salivary flow, but this effect may be reduced by the presence of fermentable carbohydrates.

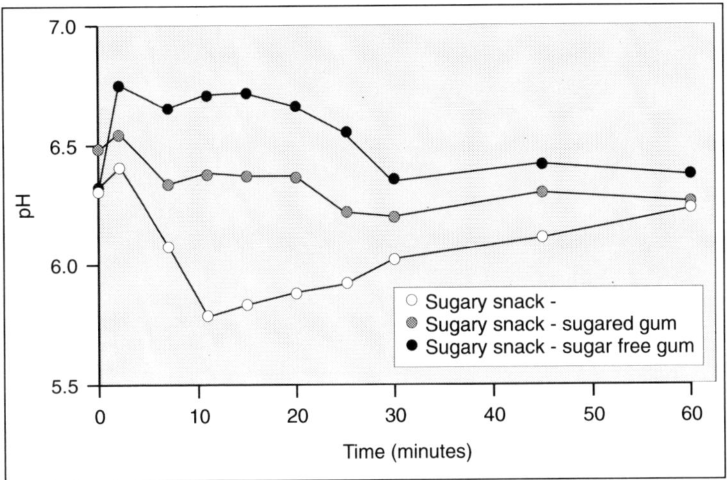

Fig. 6.4 Graph of mean plaque pH/time profiles in response to a sugary snack: challenge alone; challenge followed by sugared gum or sugar-free gum (Reproduced from Manning and Edgar, *Br Dent J* 1993; **174:** 241–244).

Recent work suggests that if sugar-containing gum is chewed after meals which contain fermentable carbohydrate it is able to exert a pH raising effect. However, this effect is less than that of sugar free gum[12,13] (fig. 6.4). It is suggested that, providing the sugared gum is chewed immediately after meals, the amount of sugar it contains provides only a small increment in the carbohydrate fermentable challenge to the plaque, and the increase in salivary bicarbonate produced by chewing sugared gum is able to overcome this increased challenge. During the remaining chewing period, after the sugar is chewed out of the gum, the salivary stimulation produced is similar to that of sugar-free gum.[13]

Chewing an unflavoured and unsweetened material such as Parafilm® following consumption of a fermentable carbohydrate gives a rapid marked increase in plaque pH (fig. 6.5) with consistent decreases in lactate and acetate and increases in the concentration of many amino acids.[14] The rise in pH accompanying chewing is closely associated with the increase in salivary flow and bicarbonate buffering (bicarbonate levels in saliva may reach 12–13 mM), but may also involve other factors including the increased supply of nitrogenous substrates for base production. The chewing of cheese, a food rich in nitrogenous substrates also elicits a rapid increase in plaque pH following sucrose rinsing (fig. 6.5) similar to that with Parafilm® ,[13] despite the pH of a cheese bolus being acidic. Not only is the pH of plaque raised to less damaging levels

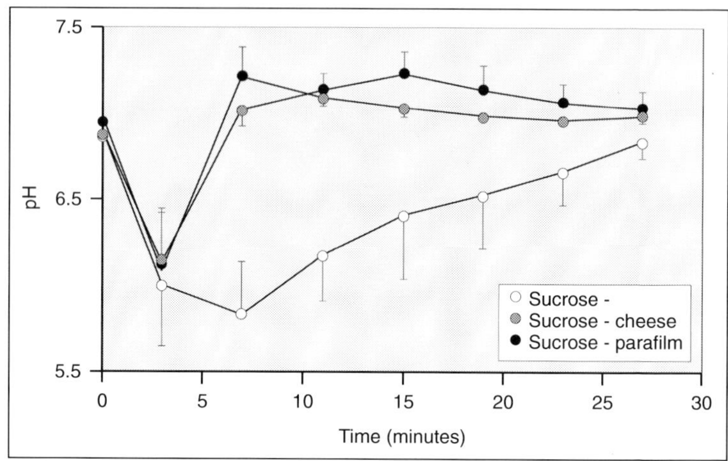

Fig. 6.5 Mean Stephan curves following rinsing with sucrose alone and following parafilm chewing or cheese chewing. Reproduced from Higham and Edgar; *Caries Res* 1989; **23:** 42–48.

in terms of demineralisation of the tooth enamel, but also the plaque fluid concentrations of strong acids fall and neutral and basic products rise. It is likely that part of the pH effect with cheese can be explained by proteolysis of cheese proteins, notably casein, but other factors may be involved including the fact that cheese is a strong sialagogue.[10] Cheese chewing also raises the plaque calcium and phosphate levels.

Similar beneficial effects have been found with chewing gum containing urea, and urea rinses. Some studies of plaque pH use the technique of chewing paraffin wax or using a urea rinse to bring the plaque pH back to normal after a carbohydrate challenge. Figure 6.6 shows the effect of a range (0.025–10%) of sucrose concentrations on plaque pH. At a low sucrose concentration, there was a small decrease in plaque pH which returned to resting values quite quickly, even without the aid of paraffin chew. However, at higher sucrose concentrations, the pH value only returned to pH 7 after a urea rinse, before the next sucrose challenge. This indicates that there was ongoing sugar metabolism in the plaque.

These results show that simple measurement of pH does not necessarily indicate the metabolic processes going on in the plaque; just because a pH value is 7, does not mean that carbohydrate breakdown is not occurring in the plaque. This implies that pH should be measured for an extended period of time. Measurement of the concentrations of

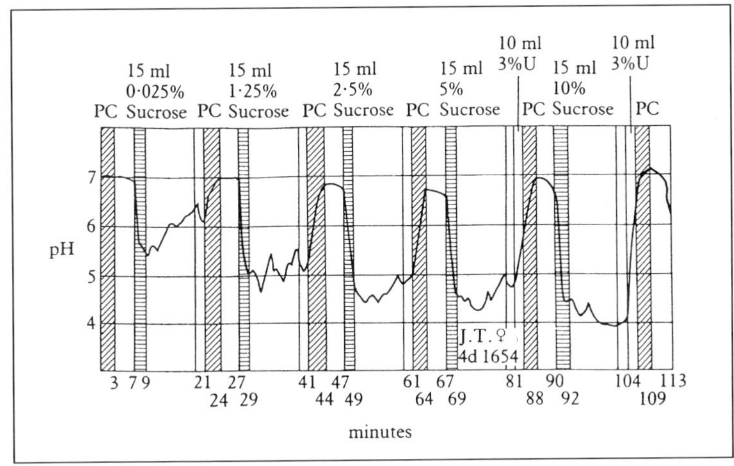

Fig. 6.6 Plaque pH measurements recorded from a pH electrode mounted interdentally in a partial denture, after rinsing with increasing concentrations of sucrose solutions (PC = chewing paraffin wax; U = urea 3% mouthrinse). Reproduced from Imfeldt; *Schweiz Monats Zahn* 1977; **87:** 448.

the acid products of metabolism gives a more direct indication of plaque activity in the mouth. Salivary pH can show a pH fall as well. For example, although stimulated saliva can raise the pH, in some studies, consumption of carbohydrates can lead to the production of enough acid from the tongue microflora to decrease salivary pH as low as pH 5. This will reduce the protective buffering of plaque by saliva.

Plaque pH in caries-free and caries susceptible patients

Caries-free subjects or those with minimal caries tend to have a slightly higher resting plaque pH, a higher minimum pH following consumption of fermentable carbohydrate and a faster return to resting levels, when compared with caries susceptible subjects. When saliva is excluded however the differences between caries-free and caries susceptible subjects are less marked and the minimum pH values reached are lower (fig. 6.7). These observations indicate the importance of saliva in modifying plaque pH and as a factor determining caries susceptibility.[15] It has been shown that plaque from caries-free subjects when compared with that from caries susceptible subjects has the ability to produce more base. These bases include polyamines and ammonia. The levels of free arginine and free lysine in stimulated parotid saliva from caries free adults has been found to be significantly higher than that from individuals with a history of dental decay.[16]

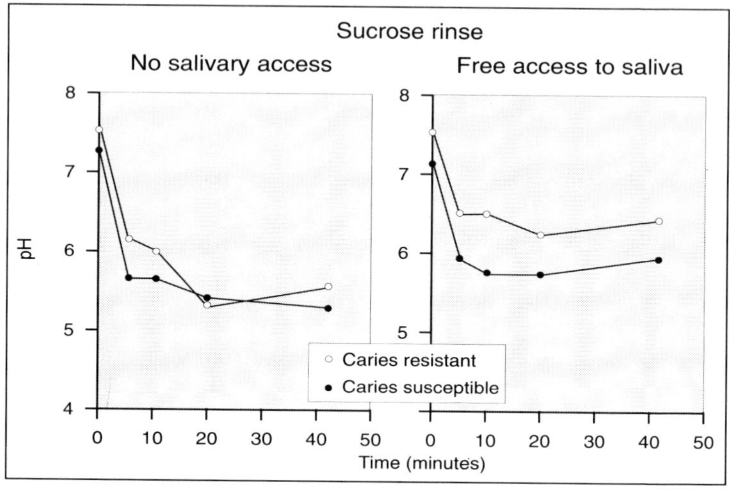

Fig. 6.7 Stephan curves from caries-free and caries-susceptible subjects when saliva is excluded (A) or not excluded (B). Redrawn from Abelson and Mandel, *J Dent Res* 1981; **60:** 1634–1638.

Clinical implications of salivary stimulation

There is a wealth of evidence advocating the benefits of stimulating saliva following eating to enhance its protective role in dental health. In recent years the use of chewing gum as a salivary stimulant has received much attention, since it has been shown to produce a continued flow of saliva during prolonged mastication.[17]

The use of sugar-free chewing gum has been found to be particularly valuable. Clinical evidence suggests that these products are non-cariogenic and when they are chewed after meals they may also reduce the cariogenic effects of other foods. Using an intraoral model system, artificial enamel lesions have been remineralised more effectively after subjects chewed sugar free gums after meals and snacks than controls who did not chew gum. Sugar-free gum has the additional benefit that it may be used over a prolonged period without increasing to a significant degree the calorific content of the diet.

Most studies involving sugar-free gums have used gums sweetened with sorbitol or xylitol. Both of these sweeteners have a significant remineralising potential, but xylitol gum has shown the stronger results. A direct comparison between sorbitol and xylitol sweetened gums in a clinical trial has suggested in a preliminary report that the caries reducing effects are greater with xylitol.[18] If confirmed, this additional effect of xylitol is probably due its antimicrobial properties.[19]

Salivary gland hypofunction

Patients suffering from xerostomia due to salivary gland hypofunction are often recommended to chew sugar-free gum, partly to relieve their symptoms but also to encourage the function of the residual secretory tissue (Chapter 4). Studies have shown that subjects with salivary hypofunction could still benefit from chewing a sorbitol-sweetened gum after a 10% sucrose challenge through the neutralising and buffering effect of the saliva produced by stimulation of their residual gland function.[20]

Summary — clinical highlights

Plaque pH is a major factor controlling the equilibrium between demineralisation and remineralisation of the teeth, the balance of which determines the progression or repair of initial caries.

Plaque pH reflects the balance between the production of acids (mainly from dietary carbohydrates) and bases (mainly from salivary urea and amino acids).

Caries susceptibility and plaque pH at different sites around the mouth are related — the higher the pH, the lower the susceptibility.

Caries-free individuals have a higher pH in plaque; this appears to result from a more active base production from salivary substrates.

Continued stimulation of saliva following a meal or snack, eg by chewing sugar-free gum, raises plaque pH and thus reduces demineralisation and favours remineralisation.

Patients with salivary gland hypofunction may, if they retain some secretory function, benefit from saliva stimulation using of sugar-free gum.

Understanding by patients of the significance of the Stephan curve and of ways by which it can be controlled helps them to know how best to look after their teeth.

Acknowledgement

We are grateful to Professor Dorothy A M Geddes, whose presentation formed the basis for chapter 6 in the first edition of this book.

References

1 Higham S M, Edgar W M. Human dental plaque pH and the organic acid and free amino acid profiles in plaque fluid after sucrose rinsing. *Arch Oral Biol* 1989, **34:** 329–334.
2 Geddes D A. The production of L(+) and D(-) lactic acid and volatile acids by human dental plaque and the effect of plaque buffering and acidic strength on pH. *Arch Oral Biol* 1972; **17:** 537–545.

3 Geddes D A. Weetman D A, Featherstone J D B. Preferential loss of acetic acid from plaque fermentation in the presence of enamel. *Caries Res* 1984; **18:** 430–433.
4 Margolis H C, Moreno E C. The effect of high pKa acids on cariogenic potential of plaque fluid (abstract). *J Dent Res* 1983; **62:** 673.
5 Kleinberg I, Kanapka J A, Chatterjee R, Craw D, D'Angelo N, Sandham H J. Metabolism of nitrogen by the oral mixed bacteria. In: Kleinberg I, Ellison S A, Mandel I D. Proceedings 'Saliva and Dental Caries' Sp. Supp. *Microbiol Abs* 1979; 357–377.
6 Curtis M A, Eastoe J E. A preliminary investigation into the identity of a major ninhydrin-positive component of dental plaque from the monkey *Macaca fascicularis. Arch Oral Biol* 1978; **23:** 421–423.
7 Kleinberg I, Craw D, Komiyama K. Effect of salivary supernatant on the glycoytic activity of the bacteria in salivary sediment. *Arch Oral Biol* 1973; **18 :** 787–798.
8 Ashley F P. Calcium and Phosphorous concentration of dental plaque related to dental caries in 11–14-year-old male subjects. *Caries Res* 175; **9:** 351–362.
9 Lindfors B, Lagerlöf F. The effect of sucrose concentration in saliva after a sucrose rinse on the hydronium ion concentration in dental plaque. *Caries Res* 1988; **22:** 7–10.
10 Lagerlöf F, Dawes C. The volume of saliva in the mouth before and after swallowing *J Dent Res* 1984; **63:** 618–621.
11 Stoppelaar J de. Urea and ammonia in saliva of caries inactive children with renal disease (abstract) *J Dent Res* 1982; **61:** 225.
12 Jensen M E, Wefel J S. Human plaque pH responses to meals and the effects of chewing gum. *Br Dent J* 1989; **167:** 204–208.
13 Manning R H, Edgar W M. pH changes in plaque after eating snacks and meals, and their modification by chewing sugared or sugar-free gum. *Br Dent J* 1993; **174:** 241–244.
14 Higham S M, Edgar W M. Effects of ParafilmR and cheese chewing on human dental plaque pH and metabolism. *Caries Res* 1989; **23:** 42–48.
15 Mandel I D. The role of saliva in maintaining oral homeostasis (Review) *JADA* 1989; **119:** 298–304.
16 Van Wuyckhuyse B C, Perinpanayagam H E R, Bevacqua D, Raubertas R F, Billings R J, Bowen W H, Tabak L A. Association of free arginine and lysine concentrations in human parotid saliva with caries experience. *J Dent Res* 1995; **74:** 686–690.
17 Dawes C, Macpherson L M D. Effects of nine different chewing-gums and lozenges on salivary flow rate and pH. *Caries Res* 1992; **26:** 176–182.
18 Mäkinen K K, Bennett C A, Isokangas P, Isotupa K, Pape JR., Hujoel P P, Mäkinen P-L. Caries-preventive effect of polyol-containing chewing gums (abstract) *J Dent Res* 1993; **72:** 346.
19 Aguirre-Zero O, Zero D T, Proskin H M. Effect of chewing xylitol chewing gum on salivary flow rate and the acidogenic potential of dental plaque *Caries Res* 1993; **27:** 55–59.
20 Markovic N, Abelson D C, Mandel I D. Sorbitol gum in xerostomics: the effects on dental plaque pH and salivary flow rates *Gerodont* 1988; **7:** 71–75.

7

Salivary Influences on the Oral Microflora

William H Bowen

In addition to containing antibacterial activities, organic components in saliva (particularly mucous glycoproteins) support the growth of many oral bacteria; variations in their relative abilities to survive on salivary growth factors can explain some of the variations observed in plaque microbial composition.[1]

Saliva and the oral microflora are major factors determining oral health. Saliva acts on the microflora by exerting antimicrobial and growth-stimulating effects simultaneously. Little is known about the growth-stimulating (nutritional) aspects of saliva, however, although the various antimicrobial systems have been studied in detail.[2] It is unlikely that any one acts alone, and the antimicrobial systems should be regarded as acting in concert.[3] The role of saliva in supplying nutrients for bacterial growth is the main subject of this chapter. Saliva may also provide nutrients indirectly through digestion of foods such as starch. It may also facilitate growth by ensuring a relatively stable pH through its buffering capacity, provision of amino acids and urea, and control of eH.[4]

Antimicrobial factors

The long list of antimicrobial factors in saliva (Table 7.1) might suggest that the mouth should not harbour any bacteria. However, these factors are part of the mouth's defence mechanisms against invasion by pathogenic bacteria, while permitting tolerable levels of commensal organisms which are not normally pathogenic. Perhaps one of the most effective antibacterial mechanisms of saliva is its washing action. Saliva harbours up to 10^9 bacteria per ml. Clearly, swallowing results in the clearance of large numbers of organisms.[5] Lack of saliva results in rapid increase in the population of micro-organisms in the mouth. Some oral bacteria are associated with bronchial pneumonia in the elderly. There

Table 7.1 Non-immunoglobulin antimicrobial factors found in saliva

	Salivary glands	Gingival exudate
Salivary peroxidase	+	-
Myeloperoxidase	-	+
Lysozyme	+	-
Lactoferrin	+	+
Aggregating factors	+	-
Histidine-rich proteins	+	-
Amylase	+	-
Anionic proteins	?	?

is growing evidence that saliva helps to control invasion of the mouth by pathogenic organisms. For example, *Streptococcus mutans*-free, desalivated rats acquire *S. mutans* from intact, infected cagemates much more rapidly than do intact, non-infected rats. A similar observation has been made with respect to Candida. Furthermore, desalivated rats infected by *Candida albicans* develop candidiasis of the mouth and oesophagus within a few weeks of being infected.

Factors which aggregate oral bacteria

Foremost among these are the mucoglycoproteins, MG1 and MG2. MG1 apparently does not interact with streptococci, in contrast to MG2.[1,6] Salivary aggregating factors are believed to be important and have been well characterised. They act by clumping bacteria together when in solution or facilitating adherence when adsorbed onto a solid phase. It is not known whether the aggregating ability or adhesiveness of bacteria is related to the abundance of glycoproteins in the mouth. The concentrations in saliva of MG1 and MG2 decline with age, which may account, in part, for the feeling of oral dryness frequently noted by the elderly.[7]

The support of bacterial growth by saliva

Saliva acts as a substrate for bacterial growth. Persons or animals who receive their nutrition by stomach tube (gavage) harbour large populations of micro-organisms in their mouths. Lactobacilli, Candida, and some Streptococci are usually absent in these circumstances.[8] However, they return in large numbers when sugars from the diet are present in abundance. Furthermore, if saliva is sterilised by passing through a 0.2 mm filter and then inoculated with plaque flora or a gingival scraping, a dense bacterial culture will develop within 1–2

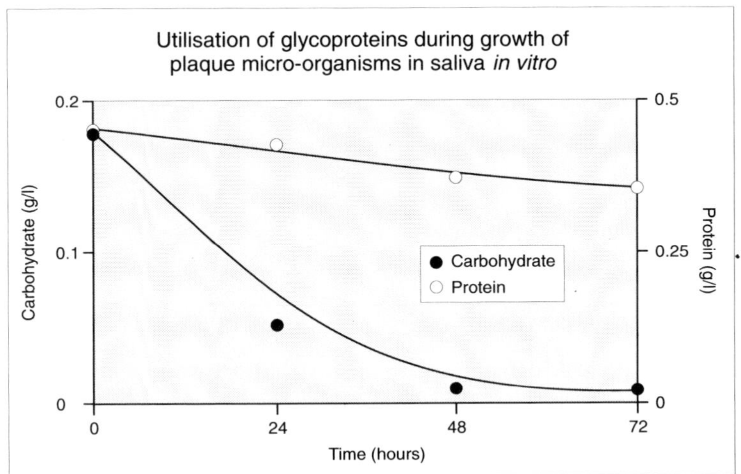

Fig. 7.1 Utilisation of glycoproteins during growth of plaque micro-organisms in saliva *in vitro*.

days. As in other microbial systems in which there is a mixture of substrates, the carbohydrates are metabolised first and then the proteins; after 24 hours incubation, the carbohydrate level in the saliva culture is low (fig. 7.1). Persons who lose salivary gland function through irradiation, Sjögren's syndrome or drugs, develop profound changes in their salivary flora. In general, increases in populations of *S. mutans*, lactobacilli, staphylococci, yeasts, and catalase-positive diphtheroids are accompanied by decreases in the numbers of *Streptococcus sanguis*, Neisseria, bacteroides, and fusobacteria. The observed changes lead to a hyper-aciduric flora are certainly related to dietary composition in addition to the absence of saliva.

Selective growth of bacteria in saliva

Saliva acts as a selective medium for oral organisms. This can be shown by inoculating plaque material into various liquids. If a common broth is inoculated, the final culture will be dominated by staphylococci, while in tap water it will be mainly Pseudomonas species. But with saliva, a typical oral microflora develops.

Incubation of plaque samples, with saliva collected separately from the major glands, suggest that the composition of the oral microflora which develops depends on the types of salivary glycoproteins present (Table 7.2). For example one strain of *Streptococcus mitior* grows better on parotid saliva while another strain grows better on submandibular/

Table 7.2 Microflora of enrichment cultures showing how different salivas select for different organisms (number of isolates)

	Parotid saliva	SM/SL* saliva
Streptococcus sanguis	4	8
Streptococcus mitis biotype 1	18	0
Streptococcus mitis biotype 2	0	18
Peptostreptococcus	4	0
Eubacterium lentum	0	24
Bacteroides intermedius	2	6
Bacteroides oralis	40	0

*Submandibular/sublingual saliva.

sublingual saliva. Most micro-organisms that grow on saliva usually have glycosidase activity. Glucose levels in saliva are too low (about 0.05 mmol/l) to explain the growth of the plaque. It is possible that it is the mucin structure which is important in selecting for particular micro-organisms. There is some evidence that gut micro-organisms have adapted to degrade, selectively, particular glycoprotein structures from the intestinal mucus. Similar differences in mucin structure might exist to explain the different types of oral flora in different individuals, but insufficient information is available. Saliva alone (in persons who receive their essential nutrition by gavage) supports a relatively simple flora; dietary constituents together with saliva are probably the most important determinants of the composition of the oral floras.

Studies investigating the role of salivary mucins

To study the role of salivary mucins in detail, pig gastric mucin has been used as a substrate. Comparable results have been obtained with human salivary mucin; however, pig mucin resembles MG1 much more than it does MG2. The pig mucin was made up into a 1% growth medium, containing no other carbohydrate, so that the micro-organisms had only the pig mucin as their carbohydrate source. The growth medium was then inoculated with different oral streptococci, and following incubation the resulting culture was examined for the growth of the inoculated strains. Various oral streptococci differed in their abilities to survive on mucin. *S. mitior* and other oral streptococci had a much greater ability than *S. mutans* to use the mucin as a source of carbohydrate (fig. 7.2). Single species were only able to degrade the complex mucin molecules to a limited extent. Utilisation of mucin was enhanced when selected pairs of strains were inoculated together (for example, a strain of *Streptococcus sanguis* and one of *S. mitior*), suggesting a co-operative action of the two strains.[9,10]

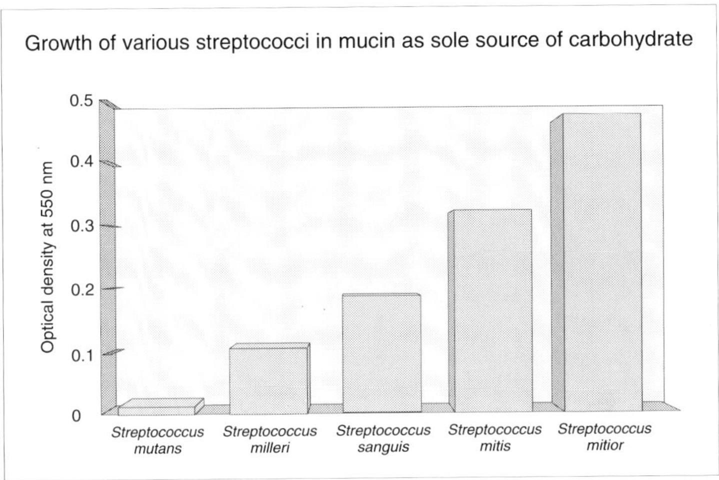

Fig. 7.2 Growth of various streptococci in mucin as sole source of carbohydrate.

The abilities of the various streptococci species to use mucin for growth seems to be related to their capacity to produce glycosidase enzymes capable of hydrolysing the oligosaccharide chains. These enzymes are seldom found in mutans streptococci, which may explain why they fail to degrade mucin to any significant extent. The inability of *S. mutans* to use mucin as a source of carbohydrate may explain why mucin-using species such as *S. mitior* are relatively dominant in early dental plaque, which is rich in mucin (fig. 7.3).[9,10] Glycosidase enzyme activities are normally determined using artificial substrates. However, data from such experiments must be interpreted cautiously with respect to the breakdown of mucin. For example, an organism may not appear to have fucosidase activity against an artificial fucose derivative, but it may still release fucose from the mucin oligosaccharides *in vivo*.

Studies conducted over decades have shown that low-molecular-weight nitrogenous constituents of saliva enhance microbial glycolysis, which leads to an enhanced termination of acid production and formation of base.[11,12] *S. mutans* and *S. sanguis* have proteolytic activity and their action on the proteins in saliva is quite distinctive. Isoelectric focussing of saliva has revealed 29 protein components with isoelectric points between pH 4.8 and pH 8.3. Following exposure to *S. mutans*, only 14 of the original components could be identified. In contrast, following exposure to *S. sanguis*, only 10 of the original protein zones were present. Furthermore, present in saliva are many free amino acids which may serve as substrates for ammonia production by oral micro-organisms.[4] *S. sanguis* can use

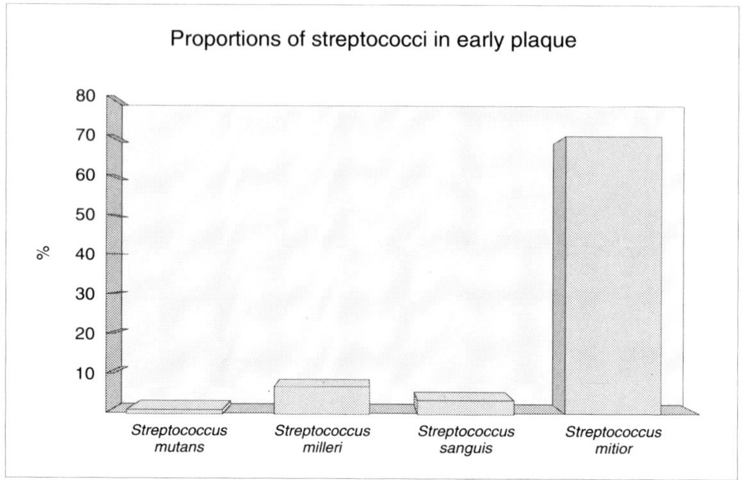

Fig. 7.3 Proportions of streptococci in early plaque.

ammonia as its sole source of nitrogen. The major base in plaque is ammonia, and the amount present varies from about 1 to 43 mmol/l. Sources for plaque ammonia include, for example, ureolysis, Stickland reaction (fig. 7.4), and the arginine deiminase system. In the mouth, arginine can be derived from the diet or the breakdown of salivary proteins. *S. sanguis* can digest arginine peptides to release arginine. The first step in the degradation of arginine (in the arginine deiminase system) results in the release of one mol of ammonia per mol of arginine. The other product in this reaction is citrulline, which is broken down to ornithine and carbamyl phosphate. Carbamyl phosphate can be further broken down to yield ammonia and carbon dioxide. The Stickland reaction may be of particular importance in dental plaque. When lactate accumulates in plaque, it may be dissipated through bacterial action involving the removal of two protons from lactate, the opening of the proline ring with the formation of d-amino valeric acid.[13]

Parallels with *in vivo* findings

It is interesting to compare the growth of oral streptococci in mucin medium with their occurrence in the mouth. In studies, monkeys were given either water containing sucrose or casein, or plain water to drink.[8,14] They were also fed by stomach tube, so that no other foodstuffs entered the mouth.

When the dental plaque was later sampled, *S. mutans* was predominant in those monkeys given water containing sucrose, while *S. mitior*

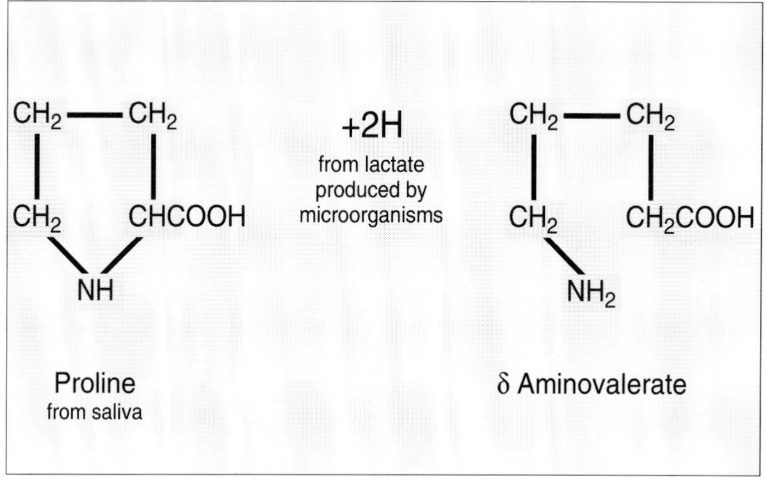

Fig. 7.4 The Stickland reaction.

was predominant in those given just water. *S. sanguis*, however, was predominant in monkeys given water containing casein (Table 7.3).

These results can be explained by known properties of the three organisms, and show that the type of energy sources available for growth are very important in determining the microbial composition of plaque. Micro-organisms can be grouped according to their preferred substrate. The results also parallel the earlier findings in culture media that streptococcal species grow on mucin, but that *S. mitior* grows better than *S. mutans* when mucin is the only source of nutrients. Ammonia is found in relative abundance in dental plaque from persons who have fasted overnight. Furthermore, d-amino valeric acid is one of the most common organic acids found in plaque. Thus, saliva alone selects for a non-cariogenic microflora with low levels of *S. mutans*. In passing, note should be taken when developing saliva substitutes that substrates are not added which would lead to an increase in the numbers of mutans streptococci.

Table 7.3 Streptococcal species as a percentage of the total microflora in early dental plaque in tube-fed monkeys (from Kilian and Rølla, 1976)

	Sucrose	Casein	Water
Streptococcus mutans	50%	0%	0%
Streptococcus sanguis	7%	48%	21%
Streptococcus mitior	4%	9%	34%
Streptococcus salivarius	2%	4%	1%

In the mouth, salivary glycoproteins are also found either as a mucosal film, or on the teeth, as the acquired pellicle. The pellicle will differ in composition from ductal saliva, as only certain components of saliva actually bind to the mucosa or tooth surface.[15] Binding of bacteria to the acquired pellicle must also be taken into account in the selection of the flora. Recent evidence has shown that bacterial-derived glucosyltransferase interacts with salivary constituents in pellicle.[16,17] Following exposure of this bound glucosyltransferase to sucrose, glucan is formed on the tooth surface which provides additional binding sites for bacteria. The major influence of saliva on plaque microbiologically can be readily observed in persons who receive their essential nutrition by gavage and those who have lost salivary gland function through disease, radiation, or use of some prescription drugs. Plaque formed in subjects who receive their diet by gavage does not lower its pH when exposed to sugar solutions.[8] In contrast, persons who have lost salivary gland function have a hyper-acidogenic and aciduric flora and may develop rampant dental caries.

Summary — Clinical Highlights

In general, bacteria can proliferate and live in the mouth. Saliva has a protective function in regulating the oral microflora, by excluding pathogens and also in maintaining the natural microflora. Saliva also acts as a source of nutrients for bacterial micro-organisms, and helps to control pH in the oral environment.

With life expectancy increasing and a growing number of elderly in the population, the prevalence of drug-induced hyposalivation is increasing. Lack of saliva can lead to susceptibility to candidiasis and enhanced virulence of *S. mutans.* The routine daily use of broad-spectrum antiseptic agents in oral products for minor oral maladies may be cause for concern. Such use appears to be based on the premise that the normal oral flora has no intrinsic value. It appears that the resident flora helps to stimulate antibody production and, in addition, helps to exclude and prevent the proliferation of potential pathogens.

References

1 Tabak L A. In defense of the oral cavity: structure, biosynthesis, and function of salivary mucins. *Annu Rev Physiol* 1995; **57:** 547–564.
2 Malamud D, Tabak L, ed. *Saliva as a diagnostic fluid.* Annals of the N.Y. Academy of Science Vol. 694. New York: The New York Academy of Sciences, 1993.
3 Biesbrock A R, Reddy M S, Levine M J. Interaction of a salivary mucin-

secretory immunoglobulin A complex with mucosal pathogens. *Infect Immun* 1991; **59:** 3492–3497.

4 VanWuyckhuyse B C, Perinpanayagam H E R, Bevacqua D, Raubertas R F, Billings R J, Bowen W H, Tabak L A. Association of free arginine and lysine concentrations in human parotid saliva with caries experience. *J Dent Res* 1995; **74:** 686–690.

5 Melvin J E. Saliva and dental diseases (review). *Curr Opin Dent* 1991; **1:** 795–801.

6 Tabak L A, Levine M J, Jain N K, Bryan A R, Cohen R E, Monte L D, *et al.* Adsorption of human salivary mucins to hydroxyapatite. *Arch Oral Biol* 1985; **30:** 423–427.

7 Denny P C, Denny P A, Klauser D K, Hong S H, Navazesh M, Tabak L A. Age-related changes in mucins from human whole saliva. *J Dent Res* 1991; **70:** 1320–1327.

8 Bowen W H. Effect of restricting oral intake to invert sugar or casein on the microbiology of plaque in *Macaca fascicularis* (*irus*). *Arch Oral Biol* 1974; **19:** 231–239.

9 van der Hoeven J S, Camp P J. Synergistic degradation of mucin by *Streptococcus oralis* and *Streptococcus sanguis* in mixed chemostat cultures. *J Dent Res* 1991; **70:** 1041–1044.

10 van der Hoeven J S, van den Kieboom C W, Camp P J. Utilization of mucin by oral *Streptococcus* species. *Antonie Van Leeuwenhoek* 1990; **57:** 165–172.

11 Bradshaw D J, Homer K A, Marsh P D, Beighton D. Metabolic cooperation in oral microbial communities during growth on mucin. *Microbiol* 1994; **140:** 3407–3412.

12 De Jong M H, Van der Hoeven J S. The growth of oral bacteria on saliva. *J Dent Res* 1987; **66:** 498–505.

13 Curtis M A, Kemp C W. Nitrogen metabolism in dental plaque. In: Guggenheim B, ed. *Cariology Today.* pp 212–222. Int. Congr., Zurich 1983. Basel: S Karger, 1984.

14 Kilian M. Rølla G. Initial colonization of teeth in monkeys as related to diet. *Infect Immun* 1976; **14:** 1022–1027.

15 Jensen J L, Lamkin M S, Oppenheim F G. Adsorption of human salivary proteins to hydroxyapatite: a comparison between whole saliva and glandular salivary secretions. *J Dent Res* 1992; **71:** 1569–1576.

16 Rølla G, Ciardi J, Eggen K, Bowen W H, Afseth J. Free glucosyl- and fructosyltransferase in human saliva and adsorption of those enzymes to teeth *in vivo*. In: Doyle R J, Ciardi J E, ed. *Glucosyltransferase, glucans, sucrose and dental caries.* pp 21–30. Sp. Suppl. Chemical Senses. Washington (DC): IRL Press, 1983.

17 Schilling K M, Bowen W H. Glucans synthesized *in situ* in experimental salivary pellicle function as specific binding sites for *Streptococcus mutans. Infect Immun* 1992; **60:** 284–295.

8
The Functions of Salivary Proteins

Donald I Hay and William H Bowen

Salivary proteins have protective antimicrobial, lubricative and digestive functions, important roles in modulating microbial colonisation of teeth and soft tissue surfaces, in providing a barrier between toxins and carcinogens and oral soft tissues, and in modulating salivary calcium phosphate chemistry. The latter is important for maintaining salivary supersaturation, so maintaining mineralisation of teeth, and also for preventing adventitious calcifications in the salivary glands and mouth. Salivary proteins also participate in the formation of the acquired enamel pellicle, a protein integument of the enamel surface that is considered to be protective, and which may influence initial microbial colonisation of teeth. Base production from basic amino-acids and peptides in saliva helps neutralise plaque acids. Collectively, these activities contribute to the functional integrity of the mouth, and provide protection against oral diseases. The mouth is a unique, highly complex, multifunctional interface between the body and its external environment. It has greater functional and biological complexity, compared to other body orifices and surfaces, including the presence of exposed mineralised tissues. The matching complexity of the proposed functions of salivary proteins is apparent from Table 8.1.

Biological activities of salivary proteins

This section presents an overview of the known biological activities of salivary proteins. These activities and the molecular mechanisms involved are discussed more completely under the headings of the respective proteins.

Control of the oral microflora

Certain salivary proteins provide important defence against bacteria, fungi and viruses.[1–6] Some of these proteins are antibacterial, controlling

Table 8.1 Salivary protein functions in the oral cavity

Oral function/activity	Associated problem	Protein function
Acts as an airway	Air-borne organisms Dehydration	Anti-bacterial systems Water-retaining glycoproteins
Speech	Need for lubrication	Lubrication system
Taste	—	Gustin
Entry-point for food mastication, swallowing	Food-borne organisms Soft & hard tissue abrasion Food toxins	Anti-bacterial systems Lubrication; mucins, statherin Toxin-neutralising proteins?
Control of indigenous & invading bacteria, fungi and viruses	Colonisation & infection Controlling pathogens and commensals Adhesion of bacteria versus their deletion	Anti-bacterial systems Immunoglobulins, histatins glycoproteins, lysozyme sialoperoxidase, lactoferrin adhesion-modulating proteins
Digestion	—	Starch & fat hydrolysis: amylase & lingual lipase
Protection & repair of soft tissues	Toxins, carcinogens, degradative proteases	Mucin-rich protective barrier film protease inhibitors — cystatins tissue growth factors?
Protection & repair of hard tissues	Enamel mineral is potentially soluble; acid-damaged enamel requires remineralisation	Biologically controlled protective & reparative inorganic environment, stabilised by statherin, acidic proline-rich and pellicle proteins
Pellicle formation	—	—
Plaque acid formation	Plaque pH control	Basic amino-acids & peptides

both the established flora and acting against invading pathogens. For example, sialoperoxidase acts to inhibit bacterial metabolism, while lysozyme attacks the cell walls of susceptible bacteria. The mucin-rich film of saliva on mucosal surfaces is considered to be a barrier against viral infections, and recently, as yet unidentified salivary proteins have been shown to diminish the infectivity of the human immunodeficiency virus (HIV).[7] It is also interesting that poor oral hygiene has been related to increased nosocomial pulmonary infections,[8–10] perhaps by aspiration of Gram negative organisms that proliferate in the mouth with reduced oral hygiene.[11]

Other proteins appear to act to control microbial colonisation of the mouth. For example, they modulate the adhesion of micro-organisms to oral surfaces. Some salivary proteins, adsorbed onto oral surfaces, evidently promote the adhesion of particular bacterial species.[12] Other proteins may aggregate some species, or block their attachment, so that they are unable to colonise and are deleted from the mouth.[5,13] In this way, salivary proteins may promote a benign commensal oral flora.

Hydration, lubrication, and protection against carcinogens and food toxins

Salivary proteins (for example, mucin glycoproteins) help form a water-retaining lubricating film on oral surfaces, so keeping the oral tissues moist and lubricated.[5] The mucin molecular structure favours the entrainment of water, so helping prevent dehydration of the oral mucosa. The mucin-rich film has also been proposed as a barrier to carcinogens and viruses, preventing their access to epithelial cell surfaces. In some rodents, food toxins, such as tannins, are neutralised by specific salivary proteins,[14] some of which are not normally synthesised and are induced by dietary tannins. Species or strains that lack these proteins, or do not adapt, are unable to grow on tannin-rich diets.

Maintaining mineralisation of the teeth

Potentially, tooth mineral is slightly soluble at pH and ionic strength values typical of saliva. Also, this potential to dissolve is greatly increased under conditions of decreased pH, such as during attack of enamel by bacterial acids, exposure to acidic food and drink, and gastric secretions. As discussed below, salivary secretions are normally supersaturated with respect to dental minerals, a property that provides important protection for the teeth.[15] Certain salivary phosphoproteins (statherin, the acidic proline-rich proteins and others) inhibit precipitation of calcium phosphate salts from saliva, and so maintain this protective salivary supersaturation.[15] In this context, it should be noted that salivary and plaque supersaturation are critically dependent on pH. Therefore, the effects of basic salivary amino-acids and peptides, and urea, as sources of base that maintains or restores plaque pH during acid production should be noted. Significant negative correlations have been found between salivary levels of these materials and caries.[16,17]

Taste and digestion

Taste has been said to depend on the presence of a zinc-binding salivary protein, gustin,[18] and the low ionic strength of saliva, compared to serum, is considered to be important for taste sensation. Saliva also has digestive activity, which in man is limited to starch digestion by amylase, and fat digestion by lingual lipase.

Genetic aspects

Because proteins are genetically determined, genetic variations will have a direct influence on the molecular structure of salivary proteins. These molecules exhibit extensive genetic variation,[19] but its role in oral diseases is poorly investigated. Limited studies of both dental caries and periodontal disease indicate a host genetic component in both diseases.

Classes of salivary proteins

Salivary proteins are synthesised in specific salivary gland cells, including serous and mucous acinar cells, ductal cells, and cells of the immune system that home to the salivary glands. In healthy subjects, only traces of serum proteins appear in glandular secretions and their presence appears to be adventitious. Serum proteins appear in higher concentrations as a result of irradiation or in Sjögren's syndrome, and are present in whole saliva, primarily from gingival crevicular fluid. Significant degradation of salivary proteins occurs in the mouth, though its extent and consequences are not well-understood. Compared to serum proteins, salivary proteins have remarkably varied properties. They range in size from ten-residue polypeptides to multi-million molecular weight mucin complexes. They are remarkably varied in their compositions, and their isoelectric points span an exceptionally wide range, far wider than serum proteins. These wide ranges in properties probably reflect a wide range of functions.

In recent years, the number of proteins detected in saliva has increased considerably. So far, some 40–50 proteins have been detected. The functions of several of these, such as carbonic anhydrase and blood group substances, is lacking or unclear. It seems likely that more proteins and protective systems will be discovered in addition to those described here.

Mucins

Mucins lack the precise folded structure possessed by many globular serum proteins. In contrast, they tend to be asymmetrical molecules with an open, randomly organised structure, consisting of a polypeptide backbone with carbohydrate side-chains. Their side-chains may end in negatively charged groups, such as sialic acids and bound sulphate, which may be important for binding between mucins and bacteria or enamel.[5] These molecules are hydrophilic and entrain much water. Such structures resist dehydration and are effective in lubricating and maintaining a moist mucosal surface. Two major mucins, MG1 and MG2,[5] have been identified. Mucins have three main functions.

Lubricating function

A feature of asymmetrical molecules like mucins is their reaction to flow. They align themselves along the direction of flow. This increases their lubricating qualities, particularly the film strength, which determines how effectively opposed moving surfaces are kept apart.

Aggregation of bacterial cells by mucin

Pure cultures of several bacterial species are aggregated by salivary and other mucins, suggesting that such species would be aggregated and deleted from the mouth. The importance of this effect is unclear, because pure monocultures do not normally occur in the mouth. Aggregation does indicate a strong interaction between the bacterial cells and the mucin, suggesting that if the mucin is bound to a surface, attachment of the bacterial cell may result. Alternatively, mucin-coated bacterial cells may be unable to attach to a surface, and such cells would be deleted from the mouth.[6]

Bacterial adhesion

Some oligosaccharides in salivary mucin appear to mimic those in the mucosal cell surface.[20] They competitively inhibit the adhesion of bacterial cells to soft tissue surfaces by interacting with reactive groups, termed adhesins, on bacterial cells, and therefore blocking them. This helps to protect the mucosa from infection. Mucins also interact with hard tissue surfaces, and evidence suggests they may mediate specific bacterial adhesion to the tooth surface. Different types of mucins are considered to fulfill these different aggregating, anti-adhesion and adhesion-promoting activities.[5]

Secretory immunoglobulins

Secretory immunoglobulins originate from immune cells which home to the salivary glands, and are produced as a host response to an antigenic stimulus.[1] This distinguishes the specific activity of the immune system from the non-specific activities of the other anti-bacterial systems. The immunoglobulins may be directed at specific bacterial molecules, including cell surface molecules such as adhesins, or against enzymes, such as glucosyl-transferase, which may be important in the biological activity of the target organisms, or in initial colonisation of the tooth surface and in plaque formation. By binding to such molecules, adhesion of specific bacteria to oral surfaces may be blocked, so selectively preventing colonisation by the affected species, or by species that share the same molecules. The potential exists, therefore, to immunise against cariogenic or periodontal disease-causing organisms. Induction of antibodies in humans against *S. mutans* was demonstrated nearly 20 years ago,[21] but practical immunisation against caries has proved difficult. The immunoglobulins may act similarly to mucins by aggregating bacteria. Although circumstantial evidence exists for complement activity in the gingival crevice, and perhaps in the overlying plaque, it seems unlikely that complement activity could act generally in the oral fluid. Thus, bacterial lysis, which requires complement activity, is not a feature of salivary antibody action.

Lactoferrin

Lactoferrin has antibacterial activity.[6] Ferric iron (Fe^{3+}) is an essential microbial nutrient. Lactoferrin binds ferric iron, making it unavailable for microbial use. This phenomenon is known as 'nutritional immunity'. A vitamin B12-binding protein has also been discovered and may act in a related way. Some organisms have adapted to the antibacterial proteins in body fluids. For example, several *Escherichia coli* strains secrete enterochelins. These molecules bind iron more effectively than lactoferrin, and the iron-rich enterochelins are reabsorbed by the bacteria. Also, lactoferrin, with or without bound iron, can be degraded by some bacterial proteases. One spirochaete, *Treponema pallidum*, can actually transport lactoferrin and use the bound iron for that bacterium's nutritional purposes. Lactoferrin, in its unbound state, has a direct bactericidal effect on some micro-organisms including *Streptococcus mutans* strains.

Lysozyme

This is one of the earliest and best characterised enzymes in the body. It hydrolyses specific bonds in exposed bacterial cell walls, causing cell lysis and death.[6] Many organisms, however, have cell capsules or other cell wall protective material, which confers resistance against lysozyme attack. Several oral organisms, including some *Streptococcus mutans* strains, do exhibit sensitivity to lysozyme in assay systems *in vitro*, but it is not clear whether the same sensitivity occurs *in vivo*, where access of lysozyme to cell walls is likely to be restricted by extracellular polymers, and especially when the cells are embedded in plaque. Some salivary proteins, and lysozyme in particular, have been said to enhance the activities of immunoglobulins, potentiating the activities of these important molecules. Thus lysozyme has been proposed as a lytic factor for bacteria to which immunoglobulins have bound, mimicking in some respects the complement system in serum. Lysozyme aggregates cell suspensions of some bacterial species.

Lysozyme and other antibacterial systems in saliva exclude susceptible invading pathogens, which are not adapted to oral conditions. This may be the most important action of the salivary antibacterial systems. However, it is difficult to assess the general clinical importance of the different antibacterial systems in saliva, as patients selectively deficient in any of these systems are rare, much redundancy appears to exist in the activities of many salivary proteins, and it seems likely that much remains to be discovered on this subject. Thus, it seems significant that subjects who are deficient in secretory immunoglobulin A (sIgA), exhibit elevated levels of the non-immunoglobulin antibacterial systems, as well as IgG, indicating that compensatory effects occur. More research is needed on lysozyme and other antibacterial substances when they are adsorbed onto the oral surfaces, where they retain activity, or present in complexes where they may exert a coordinated effect. Most studies have been restricted to the investigation of antibacterial substances in solution, rather than in the adsorbed state, such as on teeth.

Sialoperoxidase

Sialoperoxidase acts by catalysing the reaction of the bacterial metabolic product, hydrogen peroxide, with salivary thiocyanate to produce oxidised derivatives. These are highly toxic to bacterial enzymes required for energy production, and bacterial metabolic activity is inhibited. This negative feed-back control system is particularly interesting in that the activating agent, hydrogen peroxide, is produced by the bacteria, and the production of the toxic agents is highly localised and occurs close to the bacterial target.[6,22] Some micro-organisms have adapted to this control system by maintaining unusually high intracellular redox potentials.

Further study is needed to understand the balance between all these antimicrobial systems and the adaptation mechanisms of the oral microflora, both at the mechanistic level, and in terms of the quantitative effects of the systems on the oral microflora. Thus, quantitative studies[23] of the salivary antimicrobial systems showed there were no significant associations between the levels of the antimicrobial systems and measures of health status or plaque accumulation. Proportions of *S. sanguis* in plaque, however, were related to levels of some of these systems, suggesting they may affect the microbial composition of dental plaque. Another study[24] found no relationship between the growth in saliva of either *S. mutans* or *S. sobrinus* and the levels of the antimicrobial systems, suggesting that as yet unidentified adaptations, growth-promoting or growth-inhibiting activities remain to be discovered.

Histatins

This group of small histidine-rich proteins, termed histatins, are potent inhibitors of *Candida albicans* growth[2,25] and also have activity against *Streptococcus mutans* strains. Considerable advances have recently been made in understanding their anti-microbial activity at the molecular level,[26] so providing a possible basis for the design of synthetic anti-Candida and anti-bacterial analogues. The discovery of their biological activities suggests possible important functions for other small proteins or peptides, with as yet unknown functions, present in saliva. Histatin-1, which is phosphorylated, also modulates the precipitation behaviour of calcium phosphates, and histatins occur in the acquired enamel pellicle (see below), suggesting a multifunctional nature for these molecules.

Amylases

Salivary amylase is a calcium metalloenzyme, which hydrolyses the alpha (1–4) bonds of starches, such as amylose and amylopectin. There are several salivary isoenzymes. Maltose is the major end-product. About 20% of the end-product will be glucose by hydrolysis of maltotriose (three glucose residues), if the enzyme is at salivary concentrations.

Amylase appears to have a straightforward digestive function, by analogy with pancreatic amylase, and would also help clean the teeth of carbohydrate debris. But if these are its only functions, why is it also present in tears, serum, bronchial, and male and female urogenital secretions? This suggests that amylases possess as yet undiscovered biological activities in these secretions. For example, amylase interacts specifically with certain oral bacterial species,[27] and may play a role in modulating the adhesion of those species to tooth and other body surfaces. The importance of the glycosylated amylase variants is not yet clear, but the carbohydrate side-chains of these molecules may be involved in interactions with bacteria.

Lingual lipase

This enzyme is secreted by von Ebner's glands of the tongue and, together with a related enzyme that is co-localised with pepsin in the fundic region of the stomach, is responsible for the first phase of fat digestion.[28] It hydrolyses medium- to long-chain triglycerides and is considered to be important in the digestion of milk fat in the new-born. Unlike other mammalian lipases, it is highly hydrophobic and, therefore, readily enters fat globules to effect fat hydrolysis. It has been suggested that the products of lingual and gastric lipase activity help maintain the sterility of the upper gastrointestinal tract.

Cystatins

Cystatins are inhibitors of cysteine-proteases.[2,29] They appear to be ubiquitous, being present in a wide range of body fluids and tissues, and are generally considered to be protective, inhibiting unwanted proteolysis. Thus, cystatins in saliva could inhibit selected bacterial proteases, and proteases originating from lysed leukocytes. Cystatins in diseased periodontal tissue might inhibit cysteine proteases in that tissue.[30] However, detailed studies showing well-defined protective relationships in these situations have yet to be published. Several different types of cystatins have been discovered. Cystatins affect calcium phosphate precipitation and have been identified in the acquired enamel pellicle (see below), suggesting a multifunctional quality for these molecules.

Statherins

The calcium phosphate salts of dental enamel are potentially soluble under the conditions of pH and ionic strength typical of saliva. Considering that teeth are exposed to substantial volumes of saliva, far more mineral dissolution into saliva might be expected than actually occurs. The critical factor, however, is the degree of saturation of saliva with respect to the minerals which form tooth enamel. It is well established that saliva is supersaturated with respect to basic calcium phosphates, such as dental minerals.[31]

There are obvious reasons why supersaturated saliva is important for teeth. Supersaturation suppresses any tendency for the tooth enamel to dissolve, and under the right conditions, enables demineralised enamel to remineralise. Supersaturation also occurs in plaque, where it helps protect against demineralisation by plaque bacterial acids.

Theoretically, an inevitable consequence of salivary supersaturation would be crystallisation of calcium phosphate salts onto tooth surfaces. Because this does not normally happen, it was at first assumed that saliva was only 'potentially' supersaturated. Recent research, however, has identified the presence in saliva of specific phosphoprotein inhibitors of calcium phosphate precipitation.[32,33] These act by delaying precipitation from supersaturated systems, but do not diminish the protective supersaturation. Their key activities are to prevent precipitation of calcium phosphates in ductal saliva and oral fluid to maintain supersaturation, to prevent the formation of ductal stones, and to prevent calcium phosphate crystal growth on tooth surfaces.

The first of these inhibitors to be discovered was statherin (from the Greek, *statheropio* — to stabilise), a 43-residue protein, which is asymmetrical with respect to charge and composition. Several statherin variants have been identified.[34] The entire molecule is needed to inhibit primary or spontaneous precipitation of calcium phosphate, but only the first six residues — the highly acidic amino-terminal hexapeptide — are needed to inhibit secondary precipitation (crystal growth), indicating different structural requirements for these two activities.[35] Statherin is produced by the acinar cells in the salivary glands. Its survival in the mouth is difficult to determine, but it is present in significant concentrations in freshly collected whole saliva to which protease inhibitors have been added. This would seem to suggest that statherin survives for as long as the saliva remains in the mouth. The half-life of saliva in the mouth is just over 2 minutes, given normal unstimulated conditions.

Statherin is present in sufficient concentration in saliva to maintain a stable and supersaturated environment by itself.[36] But other inhibitory molecules have also been identified. Along with statherin, the main inhibitors of precipitation are the proline-rich proteins (PRPs).

The need for effective lubrication between opposing tooth surfaces seems to be rarely considered. Studies of the effectiveness of different salivary proteins as lubricants between dental enamel surfaces showed that statherin is a far more effective lubricant for this type of surface than other proteins.[37]

Proline-rich proteins (PRPs)

Inhibitors of calcium phosphate crystal growth.

Like statherin, the molecular structures of the PRPs are also highly asymmetrical.[38] Almost all crystal growth inhibition by PRPs is due to the first 30 residues at the negatively charged amino-terminal end of the molecule. In fact, the adsorption and inhibitory activity of this segment are more efficient without the positively charged carboxy-terminal part of the molecule. This large segment of the molecule differs considerably in composition from the amino-terminal 30-residue segment, indicating a bifunctional molecule. The inhibitory activity of PRPs can be explained by their adsorption onto hydroxyapatite (HA), which is considered the prototype mineral for dental enamel. They are present in the initially formed acquired enamel pellicle[39] (see below) and some investigators have found them in older, or 'mature' pellicles.[40]

Role in enamel pellicle

The acquired enamel pellicle[41] is a 0.1–1.0 µm thick layer of adsorbed macromolecular material on the dental mineral surface. It is generally thought to form by the selective adsorption of hydroxyapatite-reactive salivary proteins,[42] serum proteins and microbial products such as glucans and glucosyl-transferase.[43] The proline-rich proteins appear to be the major constituents of early pellicle, and have been reported to be present in mature pellicles.

The pellicle acts as a diffusion barrier, slowing both attack of teeth by bacterial acids and the loss of dissolved calcium and phosphate ions.[44] Although many possible candidate molecules have been proposed, the proteins that contribute to pellicle formation, and their quantitative contributions, are not yet well-identified.

Remineralisation of enamel and calcium phosphate inhibitors

The fact that early caries lesions are repaired,[45] despite the presence of mineralisation inhibitors in saliva, can be explained by the presence of the relatively sound surface layer of typical early carious lesions. This would form an impermeable barrier to diffusion of the inhibitors, which are large molecules, while being permeable to calcium and phosphate ions. If either of the inhibitory molecules were to diffuse into partially demineralised enamel lacking a sound surface zone, they might inhibit remineralisation. This could explain white-spot lesions that do not fully remineralise.

However, if the surface enamel is sound, then remineralisation of a subsurface lesion can take place even in the presence of inhibitors on the enamel surface. In fact, inhibitors may encourage remineralisation by keeping the surface pores open and preventing crystal growth on the surface of the lesion. They may thus maintain the pathways through which calcium phosphate ions can diffuse into the tooth enamel.

An additional point is that even though the pores are quite wide during certain stages of the caries attack, it is unlikely that protein inhibitors will be able to pass through the pores. Even in their degraded but still active forms, they are large molecules compared to pore size and to calcium and phosphate ions. They are also strongly charged, which may also prevent them from entering into the enamel. Thus, pyrophosphate and other small molecules used as anti-calculus agents, do not appear to affect remineralisation of early lesions.

No measurements have been made to detect whether statherin, for example, can enter the lesion. Only very small amounts would be necessary to inhibit demineralisation, and even with present techniques, such a small amount would be very difficult to recover and detect.

Calculus formation and calcium phosphate inhibitors

Calculus formation in plaque occurs despite the inhibitory action of statherin and PRPs in the saliva. This could be explained by failure of these molecules to diffuse into the calcifying plaque. Also, proteolytic enzymes, commonly produced by plaque and other oral bacteria, or derived from lysed leucocytes from the gingival sulcus, may destroy the inhibitory proteins, including the active amino-terminal segments. Plaque bacteria may produce their own inhibitors, to protect them from calcification (see below).

Calcium phosphate precipitation inhibitors and plaque

The hexapeptide from statherin and the 30-residue amino-terminal segment of PRP might be expected to occur in plaque — acting as calcium phosphate inhibitors. But analysis of large quantities of plaque has found no trace of them.[46] However, plaque bacteria themselves may produce their own calcium phosphate precipitation inhibitors, and as yet uncharacterised inhibitors have been isolated from plaque. Production of such material might be a necessary function to prevent bacterial calcification, which only seems to occur when microorganisms are dead.

Also, if crystal growth inhibitors are immobilised by being bound to gel particles, and exposed to highly supersaturated solutions, they can act as nucleators of crystal growth rather than inhibitors.[47,48] A similar situation may occur in plaque, involving immobilised inhibitors, which may encourage calculus formation.

Interaction of oral bacteria with PRPs and other pellicle proteins

Research in several laboratories has revealed some mechanisms by which microbial colonisation of the mouth may be controlled. Several salivary proteins appear to be involved in preventing or promoting microbial adhesion to oral soft and hard tissue surfaces.[12] Human acidic proline-rich proteins (PRPs) have been investigated in some detail with respect to their ability to promote selective bacterial adhesion to dental mineral. The PRPs are convenient models to illustrate this activity, although several other proteins also modulate microbial colonisation.

Clean hydroxyapatite surfaces exposed to the oral environment are known to rapidly acquire pellicles of which PRPs are a significant part. It has also been shown, *in vitro*, that PRPs adsorbed onto hydroxyapatite are strong promoters of adhesion of many important oral bacteria.[49,50] Although several organisms studied had their own profile of salivary proteins to which they adhered, many organisms adhered to a single group of proteins — shown to be the PRPs.

This work suggests that although the primary biological function of the PRPs is the control of salivary calcium phosphate chemistry, the PRPs have a secondary activity, modulation of adhesion of selected bacteria to tooth surfaces. The PRP molecule is thought to bind to tooth surfaces via its amino-terminal segment. Binding of this segment is sufficient to fulfill the primary biological role of the PRPs,[51] and leaves the carboxy-terminal region of the molecule, which has a different composition, directed to the oral cavity, and free to interact with oral bacteria.

In healthy mouths, initial bacterial adhesion to teeth is a highly selective process.[52] The resultant microflora appear to be generally benign, suggesting the possibility that host-bacterial interactions act to exclude or diminish colonisation by pathogens. In the case of the PRPs, bacteria-PRP interactions are highly specific at the molecular level. For *Actinomyces viscosus* and *Streptococcus gordonii*,[53] this interaction depends on the proline-glutamine carboxy-terminal dipeptide of the PRPs. Small changes in the glutamine structure abolish adhesion. Also of interest is the finding that PRPs in solution do not inhibit adhesion of these bacteria to adsorbed PRPs. This indicates the likelihood that the adsorbed molecules differ in conformation, compared to those in solution, and that these bacteria have adapted to recognise adhesion sites that are unique to the adsorbed PRP. Thus, adhesion of these organisms is not affected by the large excess of PRPs in saliva.[11]

Proline-rich proteins (PRPs) and statherin are present in saliva at birth (or very soon after), that is, before the teeth appear.

Summary — Clinical Highlights

An understanding of the protective mechanisms of saliva at a fundamental level is a necessary prerequisite for effective treatment of salivary gland dysfunction. Thus, progress towards modulating bacterial colonisation of oral surfaces, to eliminate pathogens, requires a good understanding of the molecular mechanisms involved in bacterial adhesion. Also, a good understanding is required of the possible interactions of various protective systems. For example, it has been suggested that the tendency to form calculus could be measured by determining the level of supersaturation of saliva, or better, in plaque, but this would not take into account factors such as possible bacterial inhibitors of calculus formation in plaque.

Synthetic saliva substitutes should, as well as mimicking the lubricating and hydrating functions of saliva, include an antibacterial system. More understanding is needed of the possible protective effect of saliva against other harmful agents that can enter the mouth, such as viruses, carcinogens and food toxins.

If a synthetic saliva is to be made containing calcium phosphate at supersaturated levels in order to protect remaining teeth, crystal growth inhibitors should be included as well. Also, there is now a real possibility of developing proteins that would bind to tooth surfaces and inhibit enamel demineralisation. Including basic amino-acids and peptides as a source for base production in plaque also seems worth considering.

Recently, significant advances have been made in developing genetically engineered multi-functional proteins, in which several of the above-noted protective activities are brought together in one molecule. Also, recent research has been aimed at introducing genes into mammalian salivary gland cells using a virus as a carrier. These approaches appear to have significant potential for alleviating salivary gland deficiencies.

References

1 Brandtzaeg P. Salivary immunoglobulins. *In* Tenovuo J, ed. *Human saliva: clinical chemistry and microbiology*. Volume II. Boca Raton: CRC Press. 1989; 2-54

2 Lamkin M S, Oppenheim F G. Structural features of salivary function (Review). *Crit Rev Oral Biol Med* 1993; **4:** 251–259.

3 Mandel I D. Non-immunologic aspects of caries resistance. *J Dent Res* 1976; **55**(Spec No): 22–31.
4 Mandel I D. In defense of the oral cavity. *In* Kleinberg I, Ellison S A, Mandel I D, eds. *Saliva and dental caries*. pp 473–491. New York: Information Retrieval Inc., 1979.
5 Tabak L A, Levine M J, Mandel I D, Ellison S A. Role of salivary mucins in the protection of the oral cavity (Review). *J Oral Path* 1982; **11:** 1–17.
6 Tenovuo J O. Nonimmunoglobulin defense factors in human saliva. *In* Tenovuo J O, ed. *Human saliva: clinical chemistry and microbiology*. Volume II. pp 55–91. Boca Raton: CRC Press, Inc. 1989.
7 Yeh C K, Handelman B, Fox P C, Baum B J. Further studies of salivary inhibition of HIV-1 infectivity. *J Acquir Immune Defic Syndr* 1992; **5:** 898–903.
8 Gibson G, Barrett E. The role of salivary function on oropharyngeal colonization. *Spec Care Dentist* 1992; **12:** 153–156.
9 Quinn M O, Miller V E, Dal Nogare A R. Increased salivary exoglycosidase activity during critical illness. *Am J Respir Crit Care Med* 1994; **150:** 179–183.
10 Wahlin Y B, Granström S, Persson S, Sjöström M Multivariate study of enterobacteria and Pseudomonas in saliva of patients with acute leukemia. *Oral Surg Oral Med Oral Path* 1991; **72:** 300–308.
11 Gibbons R J, Hay D I, Childs W C, Davis G. Role of cryptic receptors (cryptitopes) in bacterial adhesion to oral surfaces. *Arch Oral Biol* 1990; **35**Suppl: 107S–114S.
12 Gibbons R J. Bacterial adhesion to oral tissues: a model for infectious diseases (Review). *J Dent Res* 1989; **68:** 750–760.
13 Levine M J, Reddy M S, Tabak L A, *et al.* Structural aspects of salivary glycoproteins (Review). *J Dent Res* 1987; **66:** 436–441.
14 Carlson D M. Salivary proline-rich proteins: biochemistry, molecular biology, and regulation of expression (Review). *Crit Rev Oral Biol Med* 1993; **4:** 495–502.
15 Hay D I, Moreno E C, Schlesinger D H. Phosphoprotein-inhibitors of calcium phosphate precipitation from salivary secretions. *Inorg Persp Biol Med* 1979; **2:** 271–285.
16 Meyerowitz C. Caries in renal dialysis patients. *In* Bowen W H, Tabak L A, eds. *Cariology for the Nineties*. pp 249–260. Rochester: University of Rochester Press, 1993.
17 VanWuyckhuyse B C, Perinpanayagam H E, Bevacqua D, Raubertas R F, Billings R J, Bowen W H, Tabak L A. Association of free arginine and lysine concentrations in human parotid saliva with caries experience. *J Dent Res* 1995; **74:** 686–690.
18 Shatzman A R, Henkin R I. Gustin concentration changes relative to salivary zinc and taste in humans. *Proc Natl Acad Sci USA* 1981; **78:** 3867–3871.
19 Azen E A, Maeda N. Molecular genetics of human salivary proteins and their polymorphisms (Review). *Adv Hum Genet* 1988; **17:** 141–199.
20 Gibbons R J, Qureshi J V. Selective binding of blood group-reactive salivary mucins by *Streptococcus mutans* and other oral organisms. *Infect Immun* 1978; **22:** 665-671.

21 Mestecky J, McGhee J, Arnold R, Michalek S M, Prince S J, Babb J L. Selective induction of an immune response in human external secretions by ingestion of bacterial antigen. *J Clin Invest* 1978; **61:** 731–737.
22 Pruitt K M, Tenovuo J O. *The lactoperoxidase system*. New York: Marcel Dekker Inc., 1985.
23 Rudney J D, Krig M A, Neuvar E K, Soberay A H, Iverson L. Antimicrobial proteins in human unstimulated whole saliva in relation to each other, and to measures of health status, dental plaque accumulation and composition. *Arch Oral Biol* 1991; **36:** 497–506.
24 Lenander-Lumikari M, Tenovuo J, Emilson C G, Vilja P. Viability of *Streptococcus mutans* and *Streptococcus sobrinus* in whole saliva with varying concentrations of indigenous antimicrobial agents. *Caries Res* 1992; **26:** 371–378.
25 Xu T, Levitz S M, Diamond R D, Oppenheim F G. Anticandidal activity of major human salivary histatins. *Infect Immun* 1991; **59:** 2549–2554.
26 Raj P A, Soni S D, Levine M J. Membrane-induced helical conformation of an active candidacidal fragment of salivary histatins. *J Biol Chem* 1994; **269:** 9610–9619.
27 Scannapieco F A, Torres G, Levine M J. Salivary alpha-amylase: role in dental plaque and caries formation (Review). *Crit Rev Oral Biol Med* 1993; **4:** 301–307.
28 Hamosh M. Lingual and gastric lipases (Review). *Nutrition* 1990; **6:** 421–428.
29 Saitoh E, Isemura S. Molecular biology of human salivary cysteine proteinase inhibitors (Review). *Crit Rev Oral Biol Med* 1993; **4:** 487–493.
30 Aguirre A, Testa-Weintraub L A, Banderas J A, Dunford R, Levine M J. Levels of salivary cystatins in periodontally healthy and diseased older adults. *Arch Oral Biol* 1992; **37:** 355–361.
31 Hay D I, Schluckebier S K, Moreno E C. Equilibrium dialysis and ultrafiltration studies of calcium and phosphate binding by human salivary proteins. Implications for salivary supersaturation with respect to calcium phosphate salts. *Calcif Tiss Int* 1982; **34:** 531–538.
32 Hay D I, Moreno E C. Statherin and the acidic proline-rich proteins. *In* Tenovuo J, ed. *Human saliva: clinical chemistry and microbiology*. Volume I. pp 131–150. Boca Raton: CRC Press, 1989.
33 Schlesinger D H, Hay D I. Complete covalent structure of statherin, a tyrosine-rich acidic peptide which inhibits calcium phosphate precipitation from human parotid saliva. *J Biol Chem* 1977; **252:** 1689–1695.
34 Jensen J L, Lamkin M S, Troxler R F, Oppenheim F G. Multiple forms of statherin in human salivary secretions. *Arch Oral Biol* 1991; **36:** 529–534.
35 Schwartz S S, Hay D I, Schluckebier S K. Inhibition of calcium phosphate precipitation by human salivary statherin: structure-activity relationships. *Calcif Tiss Int* 1992; **50:** 511–517.
36 Hay D I, Smith D J, Schluckebier S K, Moreno E C. Relationship between concentration of human salivary statherin and inhibition of calcium phosphate precipitation in stimulated human parotid saliva. *J Dent Res* 1984; 63: 857–863.
37 Ramasubbu N, Thomas L M, Bhandary K K, Levine M J. Structural characteristics of human salivary statherin: a model for boundary lubrica-

tion at the enamel surface. *Crit Rev Oral Biol Med* 1993; **4:** 363–370.
38 Hay D I, Bennick A, Schlesinger D H, Minaguchi K, Madapallimattam G, Schluckebier S K. The primary structures of six human salivary acidic proline-rich proteins. (PRP-1, PRP-2 PRP-3, PRP-4, PIF-s, PIF-f). *Biochem J* 1988; **255:** 15–21.
39 Bennick A, Chau G, Goodlin R, Abrams S, Tustian D, Madapallimattam G. The role of human salivary acidic proline-rich proteins in the formation of acquired dental pellicle *in vivo* and their fate after adsorption to the human enamel surface. *Arch Oral Biol* 1983; **28:** 19–27.
40 Kousvelari E E, Baratz R S, Burke B, Oppenheim F G. Immunochemical identification and determination of proline-rich proteins in salivary secretions, enamel pellicle and glandular tissue specimens. *J Dent Res* 1980; **59:** 1430–1438.
41 Dawes C, Jenkins G N, Tonge C H. The nomenclature of the integuments of the enamel surface of the teeth. *Br Dent J* 1963; **115:** 65–68.
42 Hay D I, Moreno E C. Hydroxyapatite interactive proteins. *In* Bowen W H, Tabak L A, eds. *Cariology for the Nineties*. pp 71–84. Rochester: University of Rochester Press, 1993.
43 Rølla G, Ciardi J E, Bowen W H. Identification of IgA, IgG, lysozyme, albumin, alpha-amylase and glucosyltransferase in the protein layer adsorbed to hydroxyapatite from whole saliva. *Scand J Dent Res* 1983; **91:** 186–190.
45 Backer-Dirks O. Post-eruptive canges in enamel. *J Dent Res* 1966; **45:** 503–511.
44 Zahradnik R T, Moreno E C, Burke E J. Effect of salivary pellicle on enamel subsurface demineralization *in vitro*. *J Dent Res* 1976; **55:** 664–670.
46 Hay D I. Salivary factors in caries models. In: Proceedings; Chemical aspects of de/reminieralisation of teeth. *Adv Dent Res* 1995; in press.
47 Campbell A A, Ebrahimpour A, Perez L, Smesko S A, Nancollas G H. The dual role of polyelectrolytes and proteins as mineralization promoters and inhibitors of calcium oxalate monohydrate. *Calcif Tissue Int* 1989; **45:** 122–128.
48 Linde A, Lussi A, Crenshaw M A. Mineral induction by immobilized polyanionic proteins. *Calcif Tissue Int* 1989; **44:** 286–295.
49 Gibbons R J, Hay D I. Adsorbed salivary acidic proline-rich proteins contribute to the adhesion of *Streptococcus mutans* JBP to apatitic surfaces. *J Dent Res* 1989; **68:** 1303–1307.
50 Gibbons R J, Hay D I. Adsorbed salivary proline-rich proteins as bacterial receptors on apatitic surfaces. *In* Switalski L, Hook M, Beachey E, eds. *Molecular mechanisms of microbial adhesion*. pp 143–163. New York: Springer-Verlag, 1989.
51 Aoba T, Moreno E C, Hay D I. Inhibition of apatite crystal growth by the amino-terminal segment of human salivary acidic proline-rich proteins. *Calcif Tissue Int* 1984; **36:** 651–658.
52 Gibbons R J. Adherent interactions which may affect microbial ecology in the mouth. *J Dent Res* 1984; **63:** 378-385.
53 Gibbons R J, Hay D I, Schlesinger D H. Delineation of a segment of adsorbed salivary proline-rich proteins which promotes adhesion of *Streptococcus gordonii* to apatitic surfaces. *Infect Immun* 1991; **59:** 2948–2954.

Further reading

Dental caries immunisation

Smith D J, Michalek S M. Mucosal immunity and dental disease. (Concise review). *Mucosal Immunity Update* 1995; **2:** 12–15.

Handbook of mucosal immunology. (Major reference text). Ogra P L *et al.*, eds. New York: Academic Press, Inc. 1994.

Antimicrobial factors in saliva

Brandtzaeg P. Salivary immunoglobulins. (Detailed review). *In* Tenovuo J O, ed. *Human saliva: clinical chemistry and microbiology*. Volume 2. pp 1–54. Boca Raton: CRC Press, 1989.

Tenovuo J O. Non-immunoglobulin defense factors in human saliva. (Detailed reviews). *In* Tenovuo J O, ed. *Human saliva: clinical chemistry and microbiology*. Volume 2. pp 55–91. Boca Raton: CRC Press, 1989.

Salivary supersaturation with respect to calcium phosphates, and precipitation inhibitors

Hay D I, Moreno E C. Statherin and the proline-rich proteins. (Detailed review). *In* Tenovuo J O ed. *Human saliva: clinical chemistry and microbiology*. Volume 1. pp 131–150. Boca Raton: CRC Press, 1989.

Salivary factors and dental caries

Bowen W H, Tabak L A, eds. *Cariology for the nineties*. (Wide range of topics). Rochester: University of Rochester Press, 1993.

9

The Role of Saliva in Mineral Equilibria — Caries and Calculus Formation

Bob ten Cate

The importance of saliva in the prevention of dental caries is dramatically shown in patients with impaired salivary function. When, as a result of medication or radiation in the oro-facial region, salivary flow is reduced, the dentition may be completely destroyed within a short period of time. Unlike 'normal' caries, caries as a result of xerostomia is often seen at the incisal or occlusal edges of the teeth and in the cervical region.[1] This results sometimes in a chipping off of entire layers of enamel, even on the smooth surfaces (figs 9.1 and 9.2).

Saliva-pellicle-plaque

Saliva is never in direct contact with the dentition. Even at sites where the plaque is removed by the mechanical cleansing effect of the mucosa or the antagonistic teeth, a thin layer of salivary origin (the 'pellicle') covers the enamel (fig. 9.3). This layer of salivary proteins and lipids forms immediately after a surface has been completely cleaned, and it has been shown that the pellicle adheres so strongly to the enamel that it is not removed during toothbrushing or prophylaxis. The pellicle protects to some extent the enamel from severe mechanical and chemical insults, for instance imposed by acids in the oral environment.

Laboratory experiments have shown that the pellicle delays the initiation of caries and the dissolution of enamel when teeth are placed in low pH soft drinks.

At retention sites the dental plaque forms the second layer separating the tooth surface from saliva. Plaque is mainly composed of bacteria in a polysaccharide matrix. Much attention has recently been given to the liquid phase of plaque (the 'plaque fluid'), as this is the solution often in closest contact with the tooth surface. Mineral dissolution and (re)precipitation processes, as they occur during caries and calculus formation are assumed to be directed by the composition of the plaque

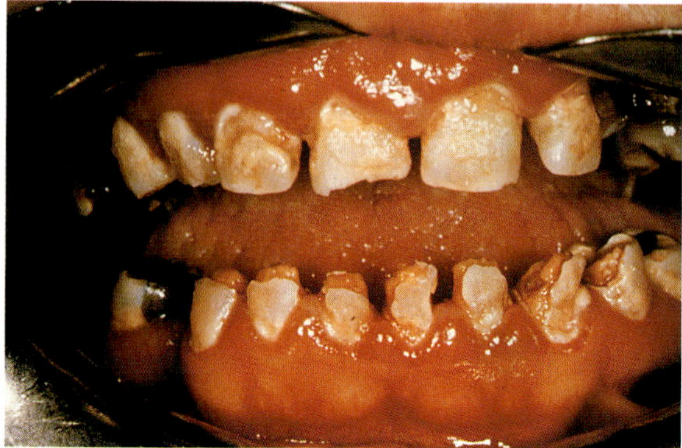

Fig. 9.1 Caries in a patient with impaired salivary function as result of radiation therapy (courtesy of Drs Jansma and Vissink, RUG, the Netherlands).

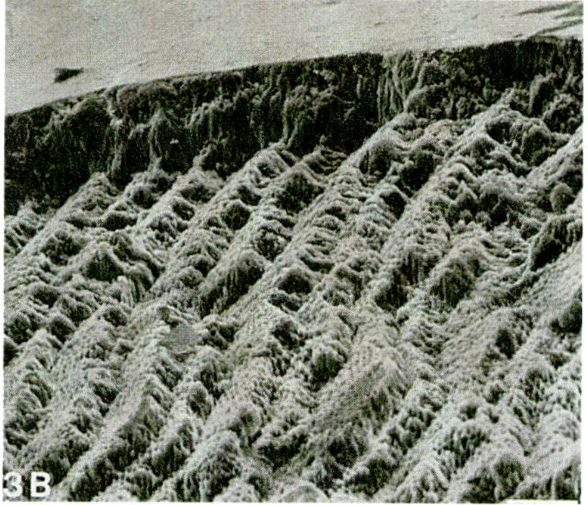

Fig. 9.2 Electronmicroscopic picture of enamel surface with radiation caries, showing the charaterictic chipping of the layers of enamel.

fluid more than by the composition of saliva, although the two are related (see below).

Enamel composition

The calcified tissues in the body are composed of a calcium phosphate mineral phase and some kind of organic matrix. The latter has various roles, such as forming the 'cement' which holds the mineral crystals together, and regulating their formation and regeneration. In enamel, the tissue forming cells (ameloblasts) secrete an organic matrix onto which crystallites are laid down. This is a process which takes place prior to the eruption of the tooth into the oral cavity. Once erupted, the ameloblasts (being on the outside of the tooth) are worn off and the fate

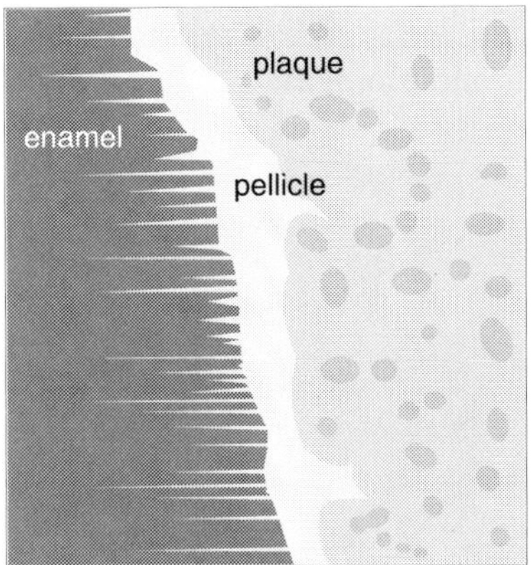

Fig. 9. 3 Schematic representation of the interface between enamel and the oral fluids, showing the acquired enamel pellicle and the plaque with bacteria and the plaque matrix.

of the enamel is no longer determined by cellularly driven mechanisms, but by the interactions between the oral fluids (the term 'oral fluid', in this chapter, refers to saliva and plaque fluid) and the enamel.

In dentine, on the other hand, the odontoblasts, being on the pulpal side, remain active and deposit so-called secondary dentine after eruption, or tertiary dentine as a result of a chemical or mechanical insult on the teeth. This can be seen as a natural defense mechanism of the body against caries and mechanical trauma. For enamel the body has to rely on saliva as a protective substance.

Saliva contains a number of components which have a specific role in this respect. The above mentioned organic constituents, proteins and lipids, form the enamel pellicle which is a diffusion barrier to acids formed in the dental plaque, and in general regulate dissolution and precipitation processes. Of similar importance are the inorganic components, especially calcium and phosphate ions. In its composition saliva possesses features similar to the other body fluids, although the degree of saturation to minerals is different.

The mineral phase of enamel consists of the calcium phosphate hydroxyapatite, HAP (Table 9.1). This mineral is the least soluble in a range of calcium phosphates which are found in nature, and more specifically in the body. Two characteristics of this substance need to be discussed in relation to their importance in the oral environment. Firstly, hydroxyapatite is very permissive in incorporating foreign ions in the crystalline lattice. These may be either positively charged (sodium, potassium, zinc or strontium ions) or negatively charged (fluoride

Table 9.1 Calcium phosphates occuring in the body

Mineral	Chemical formula	Calcium concentration (mM/l) at equilibrium at pH = 7, Ca/P = 0.1 and μ = 0.06
Hydroxyapatite	$Ca_{10}(PO_4)_6OH_2$	0.105
Brushite	$CaHPO_4 \cdot 2H_2O$	0.560
B-tricalcium phosphate	$Ca_3(PO_4)_2$	0.165
Octacalcium phosphate	$Ca_8(HPO_4)_2(PO_4)_4 \cdot 5H_2O$	0.369
Fluorapatite	$Ca_{10}(PO_4)_6F_2$	0.013 (at [F] = 0.2 ppm) 0.018 (at [F] = 0.02 ppm)

or carbonate ions). The concentration of these impurities in the tissue is influenced by their presence during its formation. These mineral modifications have either a positive or a negative effect on the solubility: carbonate incorporation makes the apatite more soluble, while fluoride incorporation makes it less soluble.

Secondly, the solubility of the apatite mineral depends highly on the pH of the environment. In an acid environment (low pH), the concentration of ions in the liquid phase surrounding the crystallites necessary to maintain saturation is higher than at high pH. pH is therefore the driving force for dissolution and precipitation of hydroxyapatite. Apart from such physico-chemical considerations other regulatory mechanisms exist, also in saliva. One example of this are 'nucleators' for precipitation: solutions which are supersaturated with respect to a given mineral do not necessarily precipitate unless this precipitate can form onto a surface. In the case of calculus formation these nucleators are the plaque bacteria, which serve to initiate mineralisation of the plaque. In enamel in contact with saliva or plaque fluid, mineral deposition may occur onto the hydroxyapatite crystallites.

In its most simple form the dissolution and reprecipitation can be described as:

$$Ca_{10}(PO_4)_6OH_2 \underset{\text{neutral}}{\overset{\text{acid}}{\rightleftarrows}} 10\,Ca^{2+} + \underset{\substack{+\\ H^+ \\ \uparrow\downarrow \\ HPO_4^{2-}}}{6\,PO_4^{3-}} + \underset{\substack{+\\ H^+ \\ \uparrow\downarrow \\ H_2O}}{2OH^-}$$

Table 9.2 Calcium, phosphate and fluoride levels in human stimulated whole saliva and plaque fluid

Saliva	Approximate concentration ranges mM/l	ppm
Calcium	0.75–1.75	30–70
Phosphate	2.0–5.0	60–155
Fluoride	0.0005–0.005	0.01–0.1
Plaque fluid[4]	**Mean (SD) values mM/l**	**ppm**
Calcium ion	0.85 (0.52)	34 (21)
Phosphate	11.5 (3.3)	356 (102)
Fluoride	0.0049 (0.0027)	0.09 (0.05)

Saliva and the Stephan curve

The mineral composition of saliva and plaque fluid is given in Table 9.2. These data show that differences in composition exist between saliva and plaque fluid, even though they are presumed to be in equilibrium. At this stage one can only speculate about the causes of this observation. Possibly the 'solid' phase of the plaque exchanges ions with the plaque fluid very slowly, which, due to its capillary nature, is never in true equilibrium with the saliva. The calcium and phosphate content and in particular the pH of these liquids determine whether enamel will dissolve (leading to caries) and whether mineral may be precipitated (which would result in calculus formation). Figure 9.4 shows the relationship between the saliva and plaque fluid calcium and phosphate levels and the saturation lines for enamel and dentine. It should be noted that the degree of saturation differs between the salivas from the various glands and with secretion rate. For instance, saliva is more supersaturated (with respect to HAP and FAP) at a higher secretion rate.

Caries and calculus formation can be explained from figure 9.4. At physiological pH, saliva and plaque fluid are supersaturated with respect to the hydroxyapatite phase of enamel. This implies that this mineral will precipitate if a suitable precipitation nucleus is available. However, after eating foods or drinks containing fermentable carbohydrates, acids are formed in plaque leading to a fall in pH called a 'Stephan curve'. When the pH is lowered, the concentration of ions needed for saturation rises, and in the pH range around 5.6 the tissues will start to dissolve to maintain saturation. The lower the pH, the faster this demineralisation. As a result, the phosphate and hydroxyl ions released will take up protons (H^+) thus slowing down or reversing the fall in pH. Consumption of foods or drinks containing fermentable

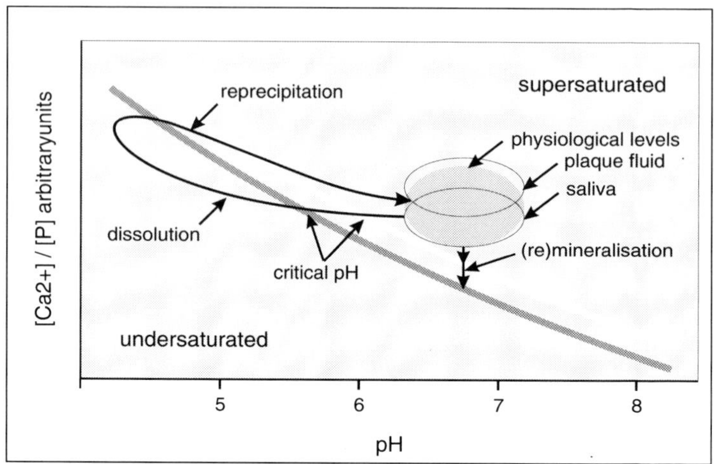

Fig. 9.4 Solubility isotherms (schematic) for enamel (lower curve) and dentine (upper curve) in relation to the levels of calcium and phosphate of saliva and plaque fluid. The change in pH after carbohydrate consumption, and the consequences for saturation of the oral fluids are also indicated.

carbohydrates also increases salivary flow; the increased buffering power of saliva, and the washing out of remaining sugars and acids from plaque, contribute to the pH-rising phase of the Stephan curve.

During the recovery phase the plaque gradually becomes supersaturated with HAP, and mineral may reprecipitate. Ideally, this occurs at the sites 'damaged' during the demineralisation. As mentioned before, the exact composition of the apatite formed depends on the composition of the solution from which it is precipitated, in this case the plaque fluid. If, for instance, fluoride is present this will 'co-precipitate' to form a fluoridated hydroxyapatite. In short, this periodic cycling of pH results in a step-by-step modification of the chemical composition of the outer layers of enamel, becoming somewhat less soluble with time. This process is known as the post-eruptive maturation of the enamel.

It has been argued that some demineralisation is beneficial because it will remove the more soluble components of enamel, rich in carbonate, which may be replaced with a fluoride-rich component making the enamel more resistant to subsequent demineralisation.

Caries and remineralisation

If the frequency of carbohydrate consumption is too high, the redeposition of mineral (during the Stephan curve) is far from complete and there is a cumulative loss of enamel substance. Then a caries lesion will be formed,

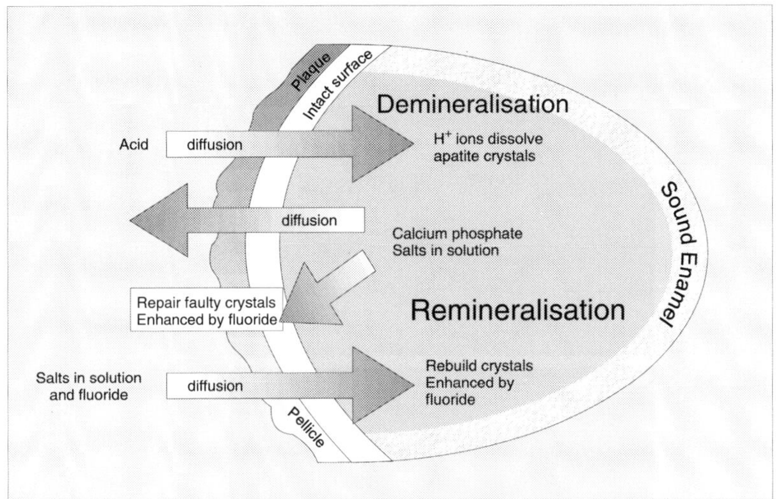

Fig. 9.5 Schematic cross-section of the enamel-pellicle-plaque interface with the diffusion, dissolution and precipitation processes occurring during caries development and regression (adapted from Featherstone, 1984).

which is often the 'forerunner' of the caries cavity. A caries lesion is characterised by a subsurface loss of mineral while the surface, due to its lower solubility, remains apparently intact. Only small pores are 'etched' in the surface layer at sites corresponding with the interprismatic regions. These enable the transport of acids into the deeper layers of the tissue and of dissolved ions out of the tissue (fig. 9.5).

Even when a lesion has been formed, saliva can play an important role in preventing excessive decay. With improved oral hygiene or other preventive measures (eg fluorides), deposition of mineral from saliva or plaque fluid may take place in favour of further tissue loss. In a laboratory model, remineralisation can be illustrated when early enamel lesions are immersed in saliva. From the radiographic pictures (fig. 9.6) the disappearance of the radiopacities is evident.

Clinically, remineralisation has been documented in a longitudinal study of drinking water fluoridation. In the Dutch Tiel Culemborg study the investigators noted that 50% of the lesions seen at the first molar buccal surfaces of 8-year-old children disappeared during the next seven years. Factors put forward to explain this finding were the further eruption of the teeth which brought the lesions out of the area at risk and in direct contact with saliva from which the remineralisation took place. A closer look at the data revealed that the lesions were seen at rather different stages. In some cases the surfaces appeared chalky and

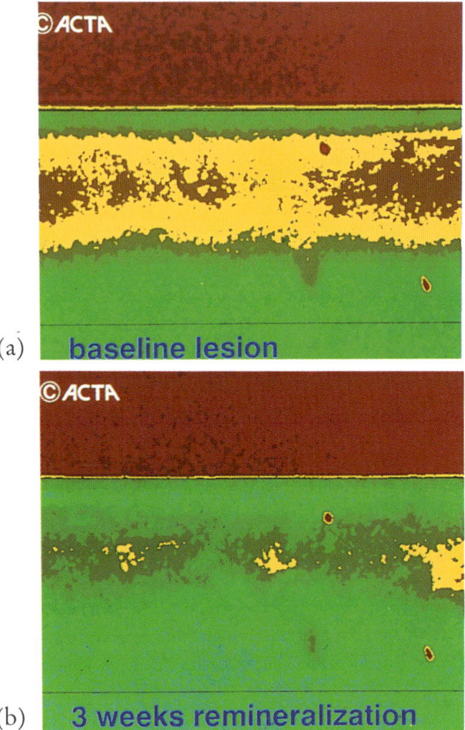

Fig. 9.6 Pseudo coloured radiographs of sections taken from lesions (a) before and (b) after a 3 week immersion in saliva, showing the disapperance of the lesion as a result of saliva-induced remineralisation (ten Cate, original data).

dull, while others were yellowish and shiny. It was concluded that the first type (found more often in the non-fluoridated town) indicated an active caries lesions. The dull appearance was due to recently exposed (non light reflecting), acid 'treated' enamel, a phenomenon also seen after the deliberate acid etching of enamel prior to placing sealants or composites. The shiny appearance of 'arrested' lesions (found more often in the fluoridated town) was due to the deposition of mineral and organic components from saliva in the porous carious enamel (fig. 9.7). With time such lesions will also accumulate dyes from food and, unless completely remineralised, eventually develop into 'brown spots'.

Calculus

Plaque is supersaturated with respect to many of the calcium phosphate minerals listed in Table 9.1. Mineralisation inhibitors present in plaque

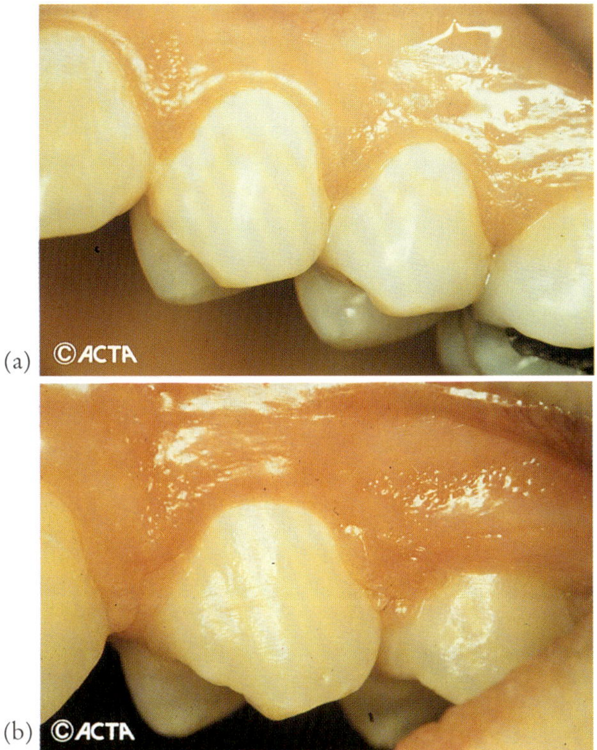

Fig. 9.7 Examples of active (a) and arrested (b) lesions (ten Cate, original data).

prevent these minerals from precipitating unless the inhibitors are degraded by enzymes or nucleators for precipitation are present. It has been shown that dead or dying bacteria (or components from bacterial cell walls) serve as nuclei for precipitation.

Unlike in enamel, where the calcium phosphate mineral is present as HAP, in calculus all calcium phosphates may be found, with the distribution of minerals being determined by the age of the deposit.

Because salivary secretions are the main sources of calcium and phosphate in the oral cavity, calculus forms most abundantly on the tooth surfaces opposite the orifices of the main salivary glands. Saliva from the parotid glands may lead to calculus formation on the buccal surfaces of the maxillary molars, while submandibular saliva may contribute to calculus deposition on the lingual surfaces of the mandibular anterior teeth. As much a difference as there is between calculus at various sites around the mouth, the variation in calculus from supra- and subgingival parts of the tooth should be mentioned. Both are formed as a result of the mineralisation of dental plaque, but in the case of subgingival calculus crevicular fluid and exudate from infected periodontal tissue substitute for saliva in providing the materials from which calculus is formed. Subgingival calculus develops from subgingival plaque, a process that is not necessarily related to a prior formation of supragingival calculus. Chemical analyses have shown that the mineral density of subgingival calculus is higher, which makes it even harder to remove by the general practitioner. The rate at which calculus forms is variable between individuals. In general, supragingival calculus forms first on the anterior teeth.

Individual variation in plaque fluid and saliva saturation and caries

Variation in the composition of the oral fluids occurs between different sites in the mouth as well as between individuals. The resulting differences in degree of saturation are very small compared to the dramatic changes occurring after acid formation in the plaque. Nevertheless, researchers have for many years been seeking to identify correlations between one individual's caries experience and his/her calcium and phosphate levels or resting pH in saliva and plaque. Recently, techniques have become available for the analysis of very small volumes (microliters), which has made plaque fluid the focus of this research. For the latter fluid a difference in degree of supersaturation (with respect to apatite) has been observed between caries susceptible and caries free subjects. These data revealed that this difference in supersaturation is primarily caused by a 0.3 unit higher pH value for the plaque fluid of the caries free individuals. Apparently, although very small, the difference in saturation has clinical implications, presumably by the difference in remineralisation potential between the types of plaque fluid. Studies to find indicators for patients at risk for caries have similarly showed that the degree of supersaturation of saliva to fluorapatite showed a high correlation with caries progression. It is argued that in particular fluoride levels in the oral fluids are an important prognostic tool.

Modifying saliva to favour caries prevention and prevent calculus formation

Caries and calculus formation are both caused by dental plaque. The most obvious direct method of their prevention would therefore, theoretically, be effective plaque removal or antimicrobial therapy. However, neither has been very effective. It seems that effective plaque removal is almost impossible to achieve. Likewise, antimicrobial approaches in caries prevention have, so far, not been very successful. Prevention therefore relies mainly on the physico-chemical mechanisms of caries and calculus, in other words once the bacteria have done their job! In the intrinsic mechanisms of caries prevention saliva has an important part, with its capacity of buffering the acid and clearing the oral cavity of foods or drinks containing fermentable carbohydrates and acids. Also saliva affects bacterial growth and metabolism.

Caries

The presence of fluoride in the oral fluids, through topical applications, dentifrices, rinsing or tablets, has a significant depressing effect on the initiation and progression of dental caries, as shown in many epidemiological and clinical studies. The smooth and interproximal surfaces benefit the most from fluoride as a caries preventive agent. During any kind of fluoride usage, fluoride is deposited at retention sites in the oral cavity. These can be porous regions (such as caries lesions) in the dentition or the soft tissues. Fluoride, when given in sufficiently large concentrations, may also be laid down on the teeth as globular calcium fluoride deposits. While in aqueous solutions pure calcium fluoride is very soluble, in the oral cavity it is surprisingly stable. This is thought to be due to the presence of a protective outer layer of the globules, formed by a reaction between calcium fluoride and phosphate and proteins from saliva. These globules may act as fluoride slow-release devices.

Saliva also serves as carrier for fluoride-ions from the various depots to the sites at risk for caries in the oral cavity. In clinical studies on the effects of fluoride dentifrices it was observed that the depot formation resulted in an elevation of the fluoride levels in plaque and saliva throughout the day. After cessation of the use of fluoride dentifrices it took about two weeks for the fluoride in plaque and saliva to return to 'baseline' levels. Now more attention is given to the patient's usage of toothpaste, which apart from brushing methods and frequency, considers what should be done after toothbrushing to guarantee optimal retention of the fluoride in the oral cavity. One advice given is to minimise the amount of water to rinse out the mouth, or to use the dentifrice (tap water diluted) as a mouthrinse. Low fluoride levels in plaque or saliva are effective in caries inhibition, because they inhibit the demineralisation of enamel and enhance the remineralisation, by an increased rate of mineral deposition. Equally important is to note that this deposition then occurs as a fluoridated apatite, which is less susceptible to demineralisation during subsequent acid challenges. The success of fluoride has initiated studies to increase the salivary levels of other 'common' ions of apatite, calcium and phosphate or the pH. Phosphate, amongst others as food additive, has been widely studied, but was never found to be very beneficial. Recently lozenges with phosphate and bicarbonate have been developed. Using these after eating elevates the pH of dental plaque above a critical level.

Many currently available toothpastes contain calcium, which is reported to have an additional preventive effects. Also xylitol is now added to chewing gum and to some dentifrices. The working mechanism relies in particular on the xylitol-enhanced salivary flow and on its antibacterial properties. The clinical effects of each of these xylitol additions are yet to be established or confirmed. Another ingredient added to dentifrices aimed at supporting saliva in its caries preventive action is bicarbonate. Bicarbonate addition increases the pH of the oral fluids which, in conjunction with fluoride, enhances mineral deposition.

Various (re)mineralising rinses have been tested. One of these is Remodent, which is a bone hydrolysate containing calcium, phosphate, many macro- and microelements and organic material. This product is suggested to be used as a stimulator of enamel maturation. Another mineralising rinse solution is based on the hydrolysis of urea which results in an increase in pH. Concerns have been expressed that the 'oral' equilibrium (in terms of de-remineralisation) is a very delicate one: too much mineralisation potential would induce calculus.

Root surface caries

Caries of the root surface has received increasing attention due to the longevity of the teeth. As a result of medication, and of diseases or surgery of the periodontal tissues, the root surface often becomes exposed to the oral cavity when the patient gets older. The tissues of the root surface are particularly vulnerable to acid attacks, and subsequently to proteolytic breakdown of the collagen matrix. Fluoride treatments have been shown to prevent this type of caries. When root lesions have formed it is now advised to first improve the local oral hygiene and give fluoride applications. This leads to a saliva-induced rehardening of the dentine. Restorative treatment can follow if indicated.

Calculus

Agents contained in dentifrices are now available which interfere with calculus formation. Crystal growth inhibitors (such as pyrophosphate and zinc citrate) are very effective in reducing the amounts of supragingival calculus, while the calculus that does form can be more easily removed.

Saliva stimulation

Stimulated saliva contains higher levels of bicarbonate buffers and is more supersaturated with respect to hydroxyapatite than resting saliva. If, after sugar intakes, saliva stimulation is prolonged (eg by chewing sugar-free gum for 20 minutes) two beneficial effects may follow: the increased bicarbonate prevents the pH of plaque from falling and thus reduces the potential for hydroxyapatite dissolution, and the increased saturation raises the potential for remineralisation of any damaged crystallites. These effects have been demonstrated experimentally using pieces of enamel from extracted teeth attached to the dentitions of volunteers, but so far have not been confirmed in a clinical trial.

Concluding remarks

As outlined above, components from saliva interact in different ways with the dentition in attempts to protect the teeth from becoming carious or from excessive calculus formation. In addition, saliva is the oral transport medium by which preventive agents are distributed around the mouth. Patients who lack sufficient saliva, suffer from many oral diseases, of which caries is only one (see chapter 4). To alleviate the discomfort they are advised to use saliva stimulants and substitutes which have the function of lubricating the oral surfaces. Most substitutes are developed for their rheological and wetting properties, and information is lacking about their level of saturation to the enamel mineral. A warning therefore seems justified that these products should be better analysed for their potential to mimic natural saliva also in its caries preventive properties.

Clinical Highlights

The arrest and/or reversal of early caries lesions is a natural and very important means of decay prevention which we can enhance by intervention.

Saliva contains calcium and phosphate in a state supersaturated with respect to hydroxyapatite. As a result, saliva reduces the dissolution of tooth mineral in caries, and replaces mineral (that is remineralises the crystals) in early lesions. Salivary hypofunction will essentially eliminate both these functions. Salivary stimulation increases its potential for remineralisation.

Fluoride in the mouth inhibits demineralisation if it is present in the aqueous phase between the enamel crystals at the time of an acid challenge.

Fluoride enhances remineralisation of early lesions by helping calcium and phosphate, derived primarily from saliva, to regrow the surfaces of partially dissolved crystals. This will produce a fluorapatite-like surface, which is more resistant to subsequent acid attack. Hence strategies which maintain the ambient level of fluoride in saliva can help control caries.

From a clinical viewpoint, a continual supply of elevated levels of fluoride in the mouth would be a very effective preventative measure.

The use of methods of delivering fluoride to the mouth (for example toothpaste or professionally applied topicals) is a very effective caries preventative measure, even in the case of severely reduced salivary flow. In fact, fluoride use becomes more essential in these patients. Because of the supersaturation of saliva, calculus formation would occur much more generally were there no inhibitors of calcification present in saliva and plaque.

Acknowledgement

Chapters 2 and 3 of the first edition of Saliva and Dental Health served as the basis for this rewritten chapter. The clinical highlights, Fig. 9.5 and limited parts of the text were copied from the first edition.

References

1 Jansma J. Oral sequelae resulting from head and neck radiotherapy. PhD thesis Rijksuniversiteit Groningen 1991.
2 Margolis H C, Duckworth J H, Moreno E C Composition of pooled resting plaque fluid from caries-free and caries-susceptible individuals, *J Dent Res* 1988; **67:** 1468–1475.
3 Sjögren K. Toothpaste technique, studies on fluoride delivery and caries prevention. *Swed Dent J* Supplement 110, 1995
4 Carey C, Gregory T, Rupp W, Tatevossian A, Vogel G L. *In* Leach S (ed) *Factors relating to demineralisation and remineralisation of the teeth.* pp 163–174. Oxford: IRL Press 1986.

Further reading

Featherstone J D B. Diffusion phenomena and enamel caries development. *In* Guggenheim B. (ed.) *Cariology today.* pp 259–268. International Congress, Zurich, 1983. Basel: S Karger, 1984.
Ten Cate J M. The effect of fluoride on enamel de- and remineralisation in vitro and in vivo. *In* Guggenheim B. (ed.) *Cariology today.* pp 231–236. International Congress, Zurich, 1983, Basel: S Karger, 1984.
Thylstrup A, Fejerskov O. *Textbook of cariology.* Copenhagen: Munksgaard, 1986.
Mandel I. Calculus formation and prevention, an overview. Compend *Contin Educ Dent Suppl* 1987;8: S235–241.

Index

Acetylcholine (ACh) 10
Acetylcholine (ACh) receptors 18, 19
Acid-stimulated salivation 32
  composition of saliva 34-37
Acinar cells 5-6
  acetylcholine receptors 18, 19
  active transport 13-14
  primary saliva production 15
  protein secretory process 21-24
  tight junctions 12
Active transport 13-14
Age-associated changes 33, 50
Aggregation, bacterial 2, 96, 109-110
Amino acid metabolism 99, 100, 101
Amylase, salivary 21, 34, 108, 112-113
Anatomical aspects 3-5
Antidepressant medication 64
Antifungal agents 63
Antimicrobial factors 2, 95-96, 111-112
Autoantibodies 57, 59
Autoimmune disease 47, 57, 59

Basolateral membrane 11, 13
Beta-adrenergic receptors 22
Bicarbonate
  buffering capacity 38, 39, 41
  in dentifrices 134
  levels 15
  plaque pH maintenance 84
  secretion 16-17, 18
Blood group substances 34, 108-109
Brushing before meals 86
Buffering capacity, plaque 82, 85-86
Buffering capacity, saliva 2, 10, 38-41
  during vomiting 31-32
  measurement in xerostomia 54, 63
  plaque pH 76-77, 83, 84-85
Bulimia 32

Ca^{2+} 16, 17-21
  mobilisation 9
  salivary content 39-40
Ca^{2+} channel 18
Calcium, addition to dentifrices 134
Calcium phosphate hydroxyapatite (HAP) 125-130
  in stimulated saliva 135
Calcium phosphate inhibitors 114-117, 130-131, 134, 136
Calculus formation 39, 40, 118, 126, 127, 130-133, 134, 136
  calcium phosphate inhibitors 116
cAMP second messenger
  crosstalk 25
  protein secretion regulation 21-24
Candidiasis
  susceptibility with xerostomia 52, 102
  treatment 63
Carbohydrate 73-74
  salivary clearance 34, 41
Carbonic anhydrase 108
Caries, dental
  calcium phosphate dissolution/precipitation balance 127, 128-130
  immunisation 110
  plaque pH 91, 92
  prevention 132-136
  root surface 134
  site-specificity 77
  variation in susceptibility 132
  with xerostomia 51, 52, 54, 63, 71, 123, 124
Carlson-Crittenden collector 55
Cheese chewing 89-90
Chewing gum
  mineral balance effects 135
  plaque pH effect 76, 88-89
  salivary clearance stimulation 34, 92, 93
  stimulated salivary flow rate 33
  sugar-containing/sugar-free 88, 89
  unstimulated salivary flow rate 34
  xerostomia management 61, 64, 93
Chlorhexidine 52, 69, 77
Cholinergic agonists 18, 19

Cholinergic antagonists 19
Circadian rhythms 7, 29-30, 37
Cl^- 14, 35
Cl^- channels 13
  Ca^{2+} regulation 16-17, 19-20
  in primary saliva production 16
Clearance, salivary 67-78
  antimicrobial function 95-96
  plaque pH 87
  with xerostomia 51-52
Collection of saliva 54-56
Composition of saliva 7, 8, 34-40
  calcium/phosphate 125-126, 127, 135
  circadian rhythms 29-30, 37
  flow rate effects 15, 16, 17, 35
Co-transport 14
Countertransport 14
Cystatins 113

Digestive functions 2, 10, 108
Drug effects
  salivary flow rate 7, 30
  xerostomia 46, 47, 48-49, 102
Dry eye tests 58-59
Dry mouth *see* Xerostomia
Duct cells 12, 15, 16
Ductal systems structure 5

Electrolytes secretion *see* Fluid/electrolytes secretion
Enamel composition 124-126
Epithelial cells 11, 12, 13
Excretory functions 2
Exocytic pathways 23

Facial nerve 3, 10
Flow rate 7
  age-associated changes 33, 50
  measurement 7, 44, 53, 60
  oral health aspects 34
  pH relationship 39
  saliva composition changes 35
  salivary clearance 34, 71
  sleep 29-30, 34, 41
Flow, total daily salivary 34
Fluid/electrolytes secretion 10, 11-21
  flow rate effects 35
Fluoride
  caries prevention 133-136
  plaque levels 87-88
  salivary clearance 69, 71-72, 74-75, 77, 78
Food intake, stimulated salivary flow rate 33, 34
Functions of saliva 1-3

G-protein coupled receptors 18, 22
Gag reflex 31
Gland size 33
Glossopharyngeal nerve 10
Glycoproteins 21, 102
  see also Mucins

Histatins 112
Histology, salivary gland 3-5
HIV 107
Hydration, salivary flow rate 29

IgA 24, 40
Imaging techniques 56
Immunoglobulins 24, 110
Inositol trisphosphate (IP_3) second messenger 18, 19
Ion channels 9, 12-13

K^+ channel 13, 16

Labial biopsy 57
Lactobacillus 97
  dip slide measurement 63
Lactoferrin 110
Lighting conditions 29
Lipase, lingual 108, 113
Lubricating function 2, 10, 107, 109, 114
Lysozyme 107, 111

Macromolecules secretion 10, 21-25
Mastication
  salivary gland atrophy with reduction 50
  salivation stimulation 31, 34
  xerostomia management 61, 63, 64
Maximum volume, salivary clearance effect 71
Microflora, oral 95-102
  in vivo substrate utilisation 100-102
  mucins adhesion/aggregation 96, 109-110
  pellicle binding 102, 117-118
  saliva as growth medium 96-97, 99-100
  salivary clearance 69-70, 77, 95-96
  salivary proteins in control 105, 107
  in xerostomia 54, 63
Microfluorometric measurements 9
Mineral equilibria 123-136
Minor salivary glands 1, 34
  anatomy 5
  collection of saliva 56
  contribution to salivary volume 35
  secretions 39, 40

'Modified' hypotonic saliva 37
Mouth moisteners 62
Mouthrinsing after meals 76-77
Mucins 96, 98-100, 107, 109-110
Mucoglycoproteins *see* Mucins
Mucous cells 5, 6
Mucous secretions 21

Na^+ gated channel 12, 13
Na^+ pump 13-14, 15, 16
NaCl, salivary composition 15
Neural control 6-7, 10-11
Neurotransmitters 10, 11
Noradrenaline (NA) 10, 22

Olfactory stimuli 32
Oral balance 62

Palatal biopsy 57
Parasympathetic innervation 6, 10
Parotid gland 1, 3, 4, 34
  collection of saliva 55
  imaging 56
  parasympathetic efferent pathways 10
  protein secretions 21
  salivary calcium/phosphate 39
  salivary volume contribution 35
  unstimulated flow contribution 43, 45
Patch-clamp techniques 9
Pellicle 2, 102, 123-124, 125
  oral bacteria interactions 117-118
  proline-rich proteins (PRPs) 115, 117
  salivary proteins 105
Peptidergic neurons 23-24
Periotron 56
pH, plaque 81-93
  critical pH 83
  elevation 83-84
  fluoride level 87-88
  minimum 83
  reduction 82-83
  resting plaque 81-82
  salivary buffering capacity 84-85
  salivary flow stimulation 88-91, 92
pH rise factors 85
pH, salivary
  bicarbonate concentration relationship 39
  calcium phosphate dissolution/ precipitation balance 126
  flow rate effects 35, 37, 41
  in xerostomia 54
Phosphate 38-40
  in caries prevention 134
  plaque pH maintenance 84-85
Physiology 7-8
Pilocarpine 19, 61-62
Plaque 123-124
  acid formation from carbohydrate 73
  amino acid metabolism 83-84, 85
  microbial composition 101
  pH *see* pH, plaque
  salivary clearance of acid 75
  salivary film 72
  site-specific demineralising/ remineralising conditions 77
  urea metabolism 83, 85, 87
Plaque fluid 127, 132
Plasma proteins, salivary 24-25, 108
Pneumonia 52, 95, 107
Primary saliva 15-16, 37
ProFlow 61
Proline-rich proteins (PRPs) 21, 114-118
Protective functions 2, 107
Protein secretion 9, 21-25, 38
  flow rate effects 35
  taste stimuli effects 36
Proteins, salivary 105-118
  classes 108-109
  digestive functions 108
  genetic aspects 108
  lubricating function 107, 109, 114
  oral microflora control 105, 107
  protective function 107
  in taste sensation 108
  in tooth mineralisation 107-108
Psychic stimuli 30
Psychological tests 58

Radiation-induced xerostomia 1, 46
  caries susceptibility 123, 124
  management 61-62
  oral microflora changes 97
Receptor-operated channels (ROC) 13
Remineralisation 39, 40
  calcium phosphate inhibitors 115-116
  plaque fluid 77
Remineralising rinses 134
Remodent 134
Renal dialysis patients 87
Residual volume, effect on salivary clearance 70-71
Rheumatoid arthritis 47, 59
Rose-Bengal test 58-59

Salitron 61
Saliva-Orthana 62
Salivary film
  buffering capacity 76-77
  salivary clearance 72

Salivary function tests 53-57
Salivary gland hypofunction 45-50
  decreased mastication-associated
    differential diagnosis 57, 58
  treatment 59-64
  see also Xerostomia
Salivary scintigraphy 56
Salivary substitutes 62, 101, 118, 135
Schirmer test 58-59
Seasonal variation 7, 30
Second messenger-operated channels (SMOC) 13
Second messengers 11
  Ca^{2+} 17-18, 19-21
  cAMP 21-24, 25
  crosstalk 25
  fluid secretion 17-18
  protein secretions 21-24
Secretory immunoglobulins 110
Secretory mechanisms 6, 9-25
Secretory tissue 5-6, 11, 12
  see also Acinar cells
Serous cells 5, 6, 21
Sialochemistry 56-57
Sialography 56
Sialometry 53
Sialoperoxidase 107, 111-112
Sjögren's syndrome 1, 47, 53, 56, 97
Sleep
  salivary bacterial count 70
  salivary flow rate 29-30, 34, 41
SM/SL saliva collection 55
Sorbitol sugar-free chewing gum 92
Statherins 107, 113-114, 116, 118
Stephan curve 73, 75, 81, 82, 93
  diet history 86-87
  salivary clearance rate effects 87
  salivary restriction effect 84, 85
  water mouthrinse effect 76-77
Stickland reaction 84, 100, 101
Stimulated salivary flow rate 30-33, 34, 43
  measurement 44, 45
  salivary clearance 71-72
Structure, salivary gland 5-6
Sublingual gland 1
  anatomy 4
  parasympathetic efferent pathways 10
  protein secretions 21
  salivary volume contribution 35
  type of secretion 3
  unstimulated flow contribution 43, 45
Submandibular gland 1
  anatomy 3-4
  parasympathetic efferent pathways 10
  protein secretions 21
  salivary calcium/phosphate 39
  salivary volume contribution 35
  type of secretion 3
  unstimulated flow contribution 43, 45
Sympathetic innervation 6-7, 10-11
Systemic disease 46, 47, 59
Systemic lupus erythematosis (SLE) 47, 57

Taste 2, 10, 108
  facilitation by saliva 37-38
Taste stimuli 32, 35-36
Tight junctions 11-12
Tooth mineralisation 107-108
Transepithelial protein transport 24-25
Transport mechanisms 12-14

Unstimulated saliva 27-30
  bicarbonate level 38
Unstimulated salivary flow rate 27-30, 43
  measurement 27, 41, 44, 45
  oral health aspects 34
  salivary clearance 71
  xerostomia 43, 45, 71
Urea
  chewing gums/rinses 90, 91, 134
  plaque metabolism 83, 85, 87

Vasoactive intestinal polypeptide (VIP) 24
Voltage-operated channels (VOC) 13
Vomiting 31-32

Xerostomia 1, 43-64
  age-associations 50
  causes 45-50
  clinical signs 51-53
  diagnosis 44, 45, 57-59
  drug-induced 46, 47, 48-49, 60, 102
  epidemiology 50
  management 59-64, 77, 93
  plaque microbiology 102
  radiation-associated 46, 59
  residual salivary flow measurement 60
  salivary clearance 71
  in systemic disease 46, 47, 59
  unstimulated salivary flow rate 28, 43, 45, 71
Xylitol
  addition to dentifrices 134
  sugar-free chewing gum 92, 134